616.994 NUL
No more cancer : a
complete guide to prevent
Null. Gary.
1039641

VE SEP 2014

D0312265

No More Cancer

No More Cancer

A Complete Guide to Preventing, Treating,
and Overcoming Cancer

Gary Null, Ph.D.

Managing Editor—Jeremy Stillman
Editor—Max W. Kortlander

Gary Null Publishing

Copyright © 2014 by Gary Null

All Rights Reserved. No part of this book may be reproduced in any manner without the express written consent of the publisher, except in the case of brief excerpts in critical reviews or articles. All inquiries should be addressed to Gary Null Publishing, 307 West 36th Street, 11th Floor, New York, NY 10018.

Gary Null Publishing books may be purchased in bulk at special discounts for sales promotion, corporate gifts, fund-raising, or educational purposes. Special editions can also be created to specifications. For details, contact the Special Sales Department, Gary Null Publishing, 307 West 36th Street, 11th Floor, New York, NY 10018 or info@skyhorsepublishing.com.

Gary Null Publishing is an imprint of Skyhorse Publishing, Inc.

Skyhorse® and Skyhorse Publishing® are registered trademarks of Skyhorse Publishing, Inc.®, a Delaware corporation.

Visit our website at www.skyhorsepublishing.com.

10 9 8 7 6 5 4 3 2 1

Library of Congress Cataloging-in-Publication Data is available on file.

ISBN: 978-1-62087-617-6
E-book ISBN: 978-1-62873-974-9

Printed in the United States of America

TABLE OF CONTENTS

Introduction

One word strikes more fear into a person's mind than any other: cancer. The disease has evolved into a national crisis that touches each and every one of us. The immense physical, mental, emotional, and financial toll that comes with a cancer diagnosis affects patients, their families, and entire communities. This year alone approximately 600,000 Americans will lose their lives to cancer, and the forecast shows no signs of improving. The latest estimates tell us that 41 percent of all Americans will be diagnosed with cancer during their lifetimes and 21 percent of the population will lose their lives to this devastating disease.[1] The vast majority of individuals who fight the battle against cancer are treated with the standard orthodox therapy, or the "official treatment." Those treated rarely question their oncologists, believing that they are in the best possible hands with their physicians' advanced education, knowledge of latest treatments, and tools of modern research.

Patients accept that these therapies have been proven safe and effective through rigorous clinical testing. We are assured that if anything really worked to improve a person's chance of survival, it could be found in the "official" medical journals and would be sanctioned by leading cancer institutions such as Memorial Sloan-Kettering Cancer Center and the Mayo Clinic. If a promising new cancer treatment comes along, we trust that it will be supported and funded by organizations such as the National Cancer Institute and the American Cancer Society. When new articles declare that a silver-bullet cancer therapy is just around the corner if we continue to obey and fund these institutions, we do exactly that with the expectation that our contributions are being put to good use in the war against cancer. Unfortunately, these institutions and their practices do not hold up under close examination. In point of fact, our belief in and support of the cancer industry and the medical-industrial complex ultimately promotes a corrupt system defined by endless greed, bad science, and appalling disregard for human life.

The most important progress in preventing and treating cancer has not come from official institutions but from those considered renegade who practice alternative medicine. Despite the well-documented success independent researchers have had using alternative therapies, they are rejected by mainstream medicine. Those presenting evidence of a cancer cure that diverts from surgery, chemotherapy, or radiation are likely to be vilified, silenced, or drummed out of the medical profession in the United States altogether.

As a result, very little progress has been made. We have been waging an official war on cancer for forty-three years and spent hundreds of billions of dollars to fund legions of scientists, physicians, nurses, and public health officials in our campaign to end this devastating affliction; yet the survival rates for most cancers—including our number-one killer, lung cancer—are still dismally low.

Cancer care in the United States has become Big Business and, like any large-scale moneymaking scheme, it is riddled with dishonesty, corruption, and deceit. It is imperative that the dark side of the war on cancer be exposed, and that is precisely what I will do in the first part of this book. I will go into great detail to present the latest information from peer-reviewed literature and many respected voices within the medical field. I will scrutinize the institutions that we hold up as authorities on cancer and take an in-depth and critical look at the treatments they support. I will highlight how our federal health agencies have completely failed us by not regulating the many carcinogens we are exposed to each day. I will also demonstrate how the medical establishment has suppressed safe and effective natural cancer therapies and, in turn, prevented millions of Americans from gaining access to scientifically proven, nontoxic cancer treatments.

In the second part of this book, I will provide the latest research on the very best foods and supplements that boost the body's immune system and can help to prevent and reverse cancer. I will explore several successful alternative cancer therapies that are practiced today in clinics across the globe, all of which are backed by high-quality science supporting their efficacy and safety. For the last thirty-five years, I have spent a great deal of time studying these treatments while visiting clinics around the world and interviewing thousands of patients. I include in this paper the treatments that I believe have the highest level of success. This is not to suggest that other holistic approaches to cancer not included are unsuccessful; I simply have been unable to verify their effectiveness.

In addition, I will present dozens of delicious and healthy recipes that can help improve and support the immune system, allowing the body to fight cancer naturally. Lastly, I will provide the inspiring testimonials of patients who, despite being told by conventional doctors that they would not survive, ultimately triumphed against cancer using alternative medicine.

PART I

THE CONTROLLERS AND PROFITEERS OF THE WAR ON CANCER

A FAILED WAR

In December 1971, with much fanfare, President Richard Nixon declared war on cancer. Forty-three years later, it's obvious that America has been fighting a losing battle. Data recently compiled by the National Institutes of Health (NIH) reveals the following:

- More than 600,000 Americans will die from cancer over the next twelve months (1,500 deaths each day).
- Approximately 1.5 million individuals will be diagnosed with cancer this year.
- Total cancer costs in our country reach $219 billion per year.
- Taxpayers spend about $89 billion per year to diagnose and treat cancer.
- About $112 billion is spent on premature deaths due to cancer.[2]

Despite these figures, our medical authorities continue to assure us that we have made significant progress in the war on cancer.

Deconstructing the Statistics

Dr. Samuel Epstein, chair of the Cancer Prevention Coalition and Professor Emeritus at the University of Illinois, Chicago School of Public Health, is an outspoken opponent of the war on cancer. Epstein's research has documented that the claims of progress by groups such as the National Cancer Institute (NCI), the American Cancer Society (ACS), and the Centers for Disease Control and Prevention (CDC) are often false and misleading. Statistics reflect that cancer rates from 1975 to 2008 increased by 15.7 percent.[3] The medical establishment has attempted to explain away the increase in cancer rates over the past four decades by pointing to smoking as the cause. In his book, *National Cancer Institute and American Cancer Society: Criminal Indifference to Cancer Prevention and Conflicts of Interest*, Dr. Epstein debunks this claim, noting that incidences of several types of cancer unrelated to smoking have risen to staggering levels during this period of time. Liver cancer rates, for example, have shot up by 177.7 percent, while cases of testicular cancer have increased by 57.9 percent.[4] Thyroid cancer rates, meanwhile, have swelled by 167.6 percent.[5]

Further, many of the statistics quoted by the cancer establishment have been manipulated to give the illusion of progress. In *Outsmart Your Cancer*, author Tanya Harter Pierce details six methods used by our health officials that deceive the public into thinking that the war on cancer has been a success:

1. Redefining "cure" as "alive five years after diagnosis," instead of using the word's real meaning, which is "cancer-free." Under this measure, a patient could still have cancer for five years and die one day after the fifth anniversary date of diagnosis but still be recorded as having been cured.

2. Altering statistics by simply omitting certain groups of people, such as African Americans, or by omitting certain types of cancer, such as lung cancer, from their calculations.

3. Including types of cancer that are not life-threatening and are easily curable, such as skin cancers and ductal carcinoma in situ (DCIS). DCIS, for example, is a precancerous condition that is 99 percent curable and makes up at least 30 percent of all breast cancers. If you deduct that 30 percent from the breast cancer success stories, survival rates are much less impressive.

4. Using early detection as a means to artificially increase survival rates.

5. Improving outcomes by deleting patients from cancer treatment studies who died before the protocol was finished, even if that was on the eighty-ninth day of a ninety-day chemotherapy protocol.

6. Using a questionable adjustment called "relative survival rate" whereby they deduct a certain number of cancer victims who statistics say would have died during the five years because of causes such as heart attacks, car accidents, and so forth.[6]

The argument that our national battle against cancer has failed because of a lack of funding doesn't hold either. As a part of the United States government's National Institutes of Health, the National Cancer Institute has enjoyed ample support from the American taxpayer since it came into its modern existence with the passage of the National Cancer Act of 1971. The NCI budget jumped from $220 million in 1971 to more than $5 billion in 2012.[7,8] Despite this sizeable increase, only a miniscule percentage of the group's budget over the years has been spent on what should be the focus of the war on cancer: prevention. Worse still, the funds allocated to help prevent this disease are drying up. In 2000, 11.8 percent of the NCI budget was set aside for prevention and in 2012, this figure dropped to a mere 3.9 percent.[9, 10]

Missing the Mark on Cancer Treatment

Not only does prevention account for a small percentage of cancer research dollars, but our national health authorities continue to downplay what may be the most important tool for cancer prevention: reducing exposure to environmental toxins. In a letter to congressional officials in 2009, Dr. Epstein and his colleagues Dr. Richard Clapp, Dr. Nicholas Ashford, and Dr. Quentin Young of the Cancer Prevention Coalition (CPC) explained why progress cannot be made without an honest discussion about limiting toxic exposure to known carcinogens. What follows are some key points mentioned in the letter:

- Exposure to cancer-causing agents such asbestos, silica, formaldehyde, benzene, chlorinated organic pesticides, and organic solvents in the environment and workplace is the largest factor contributing to the increase in nonsmoking-related cancers since 1975.
- The incidence of breast cancer has risen significantly because of environmental factors such as birth control pills, estrogen replacement therapy, toxic ingredients in cosmetics and personal care products, and routine radiation exposure from mammograms.
- Pesticides, ionizing radiation, nitrites used to preserve meats, and parental exposure to occupational carcinogens are the primary causes of the 55 percent increase in childhood leukemia.
- Hormonal ingredients in our personal care products and hormonal residues in our food have increased the incidence of testicular cancer by more than 49 percent.

- Exposure to ionizing radiation has resulted in a 116 percent rise in thyroid cancer rates.[11]

Despite ample evidence implicating environmental toxins as the primary cause of many cancers, the NCI has consistently understated and denied this connection, claiming that only 6 percent of all cases stem from environmental and occupational carcinogens. Further, Dr. Epstein's letter reveals that the NCI has ignored several calls by government officials and scientists to create a comprehensive list of carcinogens.[12]

Despite the lack of acknowledgment by the cancer establishment, there is a significant body of scientific research indicating that cancer is caused largely by environmental variables. In her 1998 book *Genetic Engineering, Dream or Nightmare?* Dr. Mae Wan Ho hypothesizes that cancer is actually an epigenetic disease, a condition resulting from "a change of the cell or gene expression state in response to the environment."[13] This is in stark contrast to mainstream medicine's view that cancer is a genetic disease brought on by DNA mutations within the cell. While the difference may seem minor to the uninitiated, Ho's theory challenges the core belief of modern medicine that cancer arises from mutations in cellular genes themselves and points to physiological stress from environmental sources as the root cause of cancer. The epigenetic theory is backed by numerous studies carried out around the world, including the research carried out by Harry Rubin, Professor Emeritus of cell and developmental biology at University of California, Berkeley.[14] The findings of Rubin and others strongly suggest that genetic mutations associated with cancer development occur *after* a cell has been transformed by physiological stressors such as chemicals and ionizing radiation.[15] Such evidence supporting an epigenetic view of cancer strengthens the argument of Epstein and many other experts that prevention should be the foremost consideration in the war on cancer. In a recent article, Dr. Ho drove home the point, stating:

> The root causes of cancer are overwhelmingly environmental, as generally recognized and hence largely preventable. Yet very little investment has gone into cancer prevention compared with the hundreds of billions spent on treatment or potential cures.[16]

In light of this information, it's clear that many of the policies adopted by the NCI have only hampered real progress from being made against cancer. An evaluation of the nation's other leading cancer organization, the American Cancer Society (ACS), turns up even more evidence of how the medical establishment is unwilling to face the reality of this disease.

Founded in 1913, the American Cancer Society (originally known as the American Society for the Control of Cancer) has become an immensely influential player in the war on cancer. Throughout its existence, the organization has come under fire for its questionable priorities; one needs only to look to the society's budgetary allocations to bring this point into focus.

In the 1970s and 1980s, I was one of very few individuals speaking out against the rampant fiscal irresponsibility and corruption that has plagued the ACS since the 1950s. In an article for *Penthouse* magazine with Robert Houston in 1979 titled "The Great Cancer Fraud," I went into detail about the dubious economics of the organization:

> The American Cancer Society had an income of $140 million in fiscal 1978, with assets totaling over $228 million; it spends less than 30 percent of its yearly income on research studies. Many feel that the American Cancer Society is largely responsible for the ineffectiveness of the war on cancer today. Contrary to the image it cultivates, the ACS doesn't conduct much of its own research but funds certain outside research.

Examining the economics of "charity," we find that 56 percent of the ACS budget goes to its staff and office expenditures (some of its executives make up to $75,000 a year).[17]

As I publicly questioned the cancer industry in articles and on television appearances, I was blasted for taking on a subject that many considered to be sacrosanct. Today, as we look back and scrutinize the activities of the ACS and other pillars of the cancer industry over the last three decades, it's clear that my suspicions about the organization have been proven to be true. In addition to their misguided priorities in deciding how to spend the vast sums they receive from generous donations, the ACS, like the NCI, has actively ignored the connection between environmental and occupational toxins and cancer. Some of the more egregious cases of the ACS actively denying this link include the following:

1971: Despite concrete evidence of the carcinogenicity of synthetic estrogen diethylstilbestrol (DES), the ACS refused an invitation to testify before Congress about the dangers of DES as lawmakers considered a ban on the substance as an animal feed additive.[18]

1977: The ACS continued to oppose regulating hair dyes that contain paraphenylenediamine, a carcinogen known to increase the risk of liver and breast cancer.[19]

1978: The ACS was officially admonished by Florida Congressman Paul Rogers for acting "too little, too late" in failing to support the Clean Air Act. Later, in 1984, the organization also balked at the opportunity to join the March of Dimes, the American Heart Association, and the American Lung Association to support the Clean Air Act.[20]

1982: The ACS narrowed its definition of what constitutes a carcinogen in such a way that the organization would oppose only those few substances that have been unequivocally shown to cause cancer in humans. The move contradicted decades of existing U.S. governmental policy, which sought to ban any food additives that were shown to cause cancer in animals.[21]

1992: In spite of the scientific evidence linking chlorinated pesticides with increased cancer risk, the ACS backed the Chlorine Institute and defended the use of the toxic spray.[22]

1994: Applying seriously flawed methodologies, the ACS published a study concluding that hair dyes pose little cancer risk, running counter to years of solid evidence establishing the carcinogenicity of hair dyes.[23]

1996: Along with other medical industry groups, the ACS lobbied the FDA to loosen restrictions on access to silicone breast implants, despite strong evidence connecting the gel found in the implants, as well as ingredients ethylene oxide and crystalline silica, with cancer in rodents.[24]

1999: The ACS dismissed the connection between genetically modified milk from cows injected with the recombinant bovine growth hormone (rBGH) and elevated breast, prostate, and colon cancer risk. Today, despite even more solid scientific evidence of this connection, the ACS declares on its website that "the available evidence shows that the use of rBGH can cause adverse health effects in cows. The evidence for potential harm to humans is inconclusive."[25]

2010: The society baselessly disagreed with the conclusions drawn by the President's Cancer Panel, which implicated environmental carcinogens such as bisphenol-A, formaldehyde, and benzene as significant factors in the cancer epidemic. The panel went so far as to admonish the ACS by calling the idea that only 6 percent of cancers can be traced back to environmental pollutants "woefully out-of-date," stating that "the true burden of environmentally induced cancers has been grossly underestimated."[26]

These are just a few illustrations of the cancer establishment's refusal to face the reality of the strong relationship between cancer incidence and exposure to environmental and occupational carcinogens. Such reluctance to discuss this association is even more surprising given the following statement taken from a 1937 article in

Time magazine written by Dr. Clarence Cook Little, director of the ACS's predecessor, the American Society for the Control of Cancer:

> Investigators have at last got a glimmering of what causes cancer. Some people inherit a susceptibility to the disease. But they do not develop cancer unless some susceptible part of the body is unduly irritated by 1) carcinogenic chemicals, 2) physical agents (X-rays, strong sunlight, repeated abrasions as from a jagged tooth), 3) possibly, biological products produced by parasites.[27]

Given the evidence, it is necessary to ask why our national cancer officials refuse to come to grips with the failed war on cancer. How can it be that groups such as the ACS and NCI remain ignorant of the environmental toxin-cancer link more than seventy years after Dr. Little brought this issue to the fore? What is it that drives these organizations to devalue the importance of cancer prevention, manipulate statistics, and write off scientific conclusions that could protect millions of people? For the answers we must take a deeper look at the major players in the war on cancer. As we'll see, the directors of this war are not virtuous independent researchers searching for a cancer cure, but rather special interests and a shady network of government agencies intent on keeping the cancer industry afloat by whatever means necessary.

Medical Deception for Corporate Gain

The Case of Sir Richard Doll

The story of British epidemiologist Sir Richard Doll not only illuminates how the medical establishment justifies its rejection of environmental toxins as a major cause of cancer; it also provides an excellent example of the powerful influence of special interests in controlling the medical paradigm. Richard Doll was a British physiologist who became the foremost epidemiologist of his time. Early in his career, Doll became the first researcher to show that lung cancer was undeniably linked to smoking tobacco. Doll also did pioneering work on the relationship between radiation and leukemia, asbestos and lung cancer, and alcohol and breast cancer. During the 1950s and 1960s, Doll was outspoken in his assertion that cancer was caused by exposure to a wide variety of toxic chemicals in our environment, ranging from asbestos to ionizing radiation.[28] In a stunning turnaround that began in the 1970s, Doll radically changed his views on environmental or occupational cancer risks and began dismissing everyday chemical exposure as the primary cause of numerous types of cancer. An influential study published in 1981 by Doll and Sir Richard Peto trivialized the occupational and environmental causes of cancer, concluding that a mere 4 percent of all cancer deaths in America could be traced back to occupational carcinogens, while only 2 percent of deaths were attributable to environmental contaminants.

These conclusions were shocking considering that Doll and Peto had previously determined that occupational exposure to carcinogens accounted for at least 20 percent of cancer deaths. With the release of the 1981 study, Doll claimed instead that a full 94 percent of cancer mortality resulted from unhealthy lifestyle habits. On further reflection, it is clear that the methodologies used in this study were flawed, resulting in inaccurate conclusions. The study examined only the incidence of cancer death rates, rather than actual cancer cases. They used only subjects who were Caucasian and under age sixty-five, ignoring the facts that cancer increases with advanced age and several minority groups are much more likely to be exposed to environmental toxins. Moreover, the results differed significantly from conclusions drawn in other studies by organizations such as the American Industrial Health Council of the Chemical Manufacturer's Association and the National Institutes of Health, which placed the percentage of cancer deaths caused by environmental hazards at 20 to 25 percent.[29, 30] Even though the Doll and Peto study does not stand up to such scientific scrutiny today, it remains a widely quoted standard within the cancer establishment.

Over the next three decades, Doll would go on to make countless unfounded and irresponsible claims that downplayed the link between environmental toxins and cancer. On many occasions throughout his later career, Doll testified as an expert witness before governmental panels and in court cases exploring cancer's connection with chemicals and radiation,[31] denying the existence of such a link, and thus preventing injured workers from being compensated for damage by asbestos, radiation, and other carcinogens.

What was behind Richard Doll's dramatic change of opinion? It would come to light in 2006—one year after his death—that Doll was being handsomely compensated by a collection of corporate interests that stood to lose many millions of dollars if the truth about their cancer-causing products were made public. Not surprisingly, the scientist's reversal of opinion on the link between environmental carcinogens and cancer coincided perfectly with the start of his clandestine career as an industry consultant.

Looking back, we can see many examples of how Doll worked diligently for special interests. In one case, Doll wrote to an Australian Royal Commission investigating the carcinogenicity of the notorious Agent Orange herbicide manufactured by Monsanto and sprayed by U.S. warplanes during the Vietnam War.[32] Though research suggested a link existed between Agent Orange and cancer, Sir Richard's missive flatly denied any connection. As it turned out, Doll had been working as a consultant to Monsanto at the time. Documents indicate that Doll earned between $1,000 and $1,500 per day in his long tenure with Monsanto, which stretched from 1976 to at least 2000.[33]

Monsanto was not the only company to sully Doll's scientific credibility. Documents indicate that in one case Doll received tens of thousands of dollars from chemical giants Dow Chemicals and ICI as well as the Chemical Manufacturers' Association.[34] In an apparent quid pro quo agreement, Doll publicly defended the use of the carcinogenic plastic ingredient vinyl chloride, denying its connection to an increased risk of brain and liver cancer. As a powerful and influential scientist, Doll's defense allowed the chemical industry to justify the manufacture of the disease-causing agent for years afterward, and helped stymie cancer victims exposed to vinyl chloride from seeking legal damages.[35] Vinyl chloride was finally banned in 1978 after an Italian scientist proved the cancer connection definitively.

Doll's work on asbestos may have represented his turning point from impartial scientist to industry spokesman. In 1954, Doll and a colleague began investigating asbestos hazards in workers at the Turner & Newall plant in Manchester, England, and found that exposed workers developed lung cancer at ten times the rate of workers who were not in contact with the chemical. The company successfully blocked publication of these findings. Shortly thereafter, in a bizarre shift, Doll began to publicly assert that asbestos, in fact, was only minimally harmful. Doll was criticized in 1985 by the U.K. Society for the Prevention of Asbestos and Industrial Disease for distorting data to suggest that only 1 out of every 100,000 people exposed to undamaged asbestos in the workplace was at risk of developing cancer, when the true threat was, in fact, far greater.[36] Ultimately, Doll became a paid consultant for Turner & Newall.[37] In 2000, Doll admitted in a deposition that a £50,000 donation by the asbestos company Turner & Newall to Green College in Oxford (where Doll served as a professor and administrator) was "in recognition of all the work I had done for them."[38]

The story of Sir Richard Doll is a perfect illustration of how corporate profiteers have co-opted science in the United States. Thoroughly in thrall to the interests of chemical manufacturers and others, Doll spent decades as a leading authority on cancer, minimizing the real risks surrounding environmental pollution. The adverse public health consequences of such blatant manipulation of scientific evidence are immeasurable, and have likely affected millions of people across the globe. Ironically, a few years before his death, Doll seemed to have another dramatic change of heart. The scientist acknowledged in 2002 that the majority of cancers that are unrelated to smoking and hormones "are caused by exposure to chemicals, often environmental."[39]

A Critical Look at the American Cancer Society

The egregious medical deception on the part of Sir Richard Doll and his industry backers is far from exceptional. We don't have to look far to find heavy corporate manipulation of public cancer policy. One of the greatest exemplars of this collusive relationship is the American Cancer Society (ACS).

The American Cancer Society started out as the American Society for the Control of Cancer in 1913, an organization composed primarily of top physicians to promote dissemination of current information about the development and treatment of cancer. In the 1940s, Mary Lasker and her husband—the influential advertising executive, Albert Lasker—transformed the group into the American Cancer Society. Control shifted from the group's dedicated physicians to representatives of industry as the ACS developed into a fundraising and research powerhouse.

My investigations were among the first to call attention to the serious conflicts of interest that infected the ACS. More than thirty years ago, I reported that "approximately 70 percent of the ACS's meager research budget goes to support research that is carried on by institutions with which the board of directors affiliate."[40] The truth is that, for over half a century, a collection of special interests has figured prominently in the decision making that goes on at the ACS.

Devra Davis explains in *The Secret History of the War on Cancer* how, throughout the 1940s, the leadership at the ACS was infiltrated by a group of powerful corporate leaders. Among the business moguls that rose to positions of power in the ACS was Elmer Bobst, the CEO of the pharmaceutical company Warner Chilcott. Albert Lasker, also involved in the corporate takeover, was a pioneer in the field of marketing. It was Lasker who got thousands of American women hooked on cigarettes after crafting a slogan for the American Tobacco Company that declared, "Reach for a Lucky instead of a sweet."[41] Corporate control of the ACS became further entrenched during the next few decades as industry barons such as W.B. Lewis, who served as the vice president for tobacco company Liggett and Myers, gained influential positions within the organization.

Over the next couple of decades, the evidence linking smoking cigarettes and lung cancer was increasingly incontestable,[42] yet many worked to keep such information from reaching the public. Former ACS president Ashbel Williams openly admitted to the ACS board's resistance to sharing evidence of the serious cancer risks posed by cigarettes. Williams commented during one interview, "Our early efforts were bottled up. . . . We accomplished nothing. There were two Board members, one from Louisville, Kentucky, who stymied any assertive statements by the Society."[43]

In an ironic shift from the 1960s, the ACS has come to emphasize smoking and aging of the population as the principal causes of cancer while largely ignoring the irrefutable and ever-expanding body of research associating the nation's cancer epidemic with environmental and occupational carcinogens. To make sense of this institutional denial, one must simply examine the organization's more recent corporate alliances. The ACS receives sizeable donations from corporations that either sell carcinogenic products or stand to profit from the cancer epidemic itself. According to a report by Samuel Epstein in 2010, companies that have donated more than $100,000 to the ACS in previous years include:

- Petrochemical companies (DuPont, BP, and Pennzoil)
- Industrial waste companies (BFI Waste Systems)
- Junk food companies (Wendy's International, McDonald's, Unilever/Best Foods, and Coca-Cola)
- Big Pharma (AstraZeneca, Bristol-Myers Squibb, GlaxoSmithKline, Merck & Company, and Novartis)
- Biotech companies (Amgen and Genentech)
- Cosmetic companies (Christian Dior, Avon, Revlon, Elizabeth Arden, and Estée Lauder)
- Auto companies (Nissan and General Motors)[44]

The influence held by special interests in dictating ACS's policy is also evident upon reviewing the organization's board of trustees.

Described as the world's wealthiest nonprofit[45], the ACS Foundation was started in 1992 to solicit large contributions from wealthy donors. Those who have sat on the foundation's board have strong ties to various sectors of American Big Business. Former board members include Alan Gevertzen, the former chair of the board of contracting giant Boeing; Sumner M. Redstone, media tycoon and majority owner of CBS News and Viacom; and Gordon Binder, former chair and CEO of the world's largest independent biotechnology company, Amgen.[46]

Despite its nonprofit status, the ACS has amassed considerable wealth over the years through donations from both public and private enterprises. In 1988, a paltry 26 percent of the society's $400 million budget went toward medical research and programs, while the remaining funds were put toward so-called "operating expenses"—60 percent of which were allotted for "generous salaries, pensions, executive benefits, and overhead."[47]

Despite the glaring conflicts of interest and misallocation of resources that continue to characterize the ACS to this day, the funds flowing into group have increased tremendously since the 1980s, exceeding $1.33 billion in 2009.[48] That same year, the CEO of the American Cancer Society, John Seffrin, earned $914,906,[49] and two former ACS officials were given even more generous payouts: the former National Vice President of Divisional Services, William Barram, and the retired Deputy CEO, Donald Thomas, earned $1,550,705 and $1,407,719, respectively.[50]

Questioning the National Cancer Institute

Since its inception in 1937, the National Cancer Institute has enjoyed generous support from the American taxpayer yet under its watch, overall cancer rates have actually increased. It is imperative that we examine the reasons behind this organization's failure to protect the

American people. As with the ACS, it is undeniable that many NCI policies have been shaped by special interests.

The NCI has a history of close ties with groups that manufacture or promote cancer-causing products. In 1971, at the beginning of Nixon's War on Cancer, the President's Cancer Panel was created to oversee the NCI as the president's watchdog. The first chair of the President's Cancer Panel was Benno C. Schmidt, partner of the wealthy Jock Whitney in one of the first venture capital firms, J. H. Whitney & Co., which invested widely in chemical and pharmaceutical companies. In addition to having a cozy relationship with the oil, steel, and chemical industries, Schmidt served as the executive of a pharmaceutical company and served on many company boards of directors.[51] Schmidt was responsible for firing NCI director Carl Baker and replacing him with Dr. Frank Rauscher, a virologist. Dr. Rauscher was NCI director from 1971 to 1976, then moved on to become the Senior Vice President of the ACS. His tenure at the ACS ended in 1988, when he took on the role of executive director of the Thermal Insulation Manufacturers Association, known for its endorsement of home decorating products such as fiberglass, which contain carcinogens such as styrene and formaldehyde.[52] When Benno Schmidt's tenure ended as chair of the President's Cancer Panel he was replaced by Armand Hammer, the wealthy industrialist who presided over one of the country's largest chemical companies as the chair of the Occidental Petroleum Corporation.[53] The record reflects that under the leadership of these men, the NCI prioritized the creation of ineffective, costly, and toxic cancer drugs while neglecting to emphasize the importance of prevention.

Let's take a look at a few more conflicts of interest within the NCI that have propped up the cancer industry at the expense of Americans' health.

- 1992: Funded by American taxpayer dollars, the NCI sponsored research by Bristol-Myers Squibb to develop what would become the breast cancer chemotherapy drug Taxol. Bristol-Myers Squibb would go on to earn billions off Taxol, selling it to consumers at $4.87 per milligram, or twenty times the cost of production.[54] A study published in *The New England Journal of Medicine* in 2007 exposes that Taxol is wholly ineffective in treating the most common form of breast cancer, estrogen receptor negative.[55] This translates to around 20,000 American women unnecessarily suffering debilitating side effects from a useless chemotherapy treatment each year.[56]

- 1995: Harold Varmus, the head of the National Institutes of Health (who currently serves as the director of the NCI), further opened the doors to pharmaceutical industry influence by granting NCI employees free license to consult with the cancer drug industry.[57] Varmus also would later go on to receive a compensation package of $2.7 million. This generous salary, according to the Charity Rating Guide & Watchdog Report, was the "highest compensation of directors in over 500 major nonprofit organizations ever monitored."[58]

- 1997: After spending millions to sponsor the NCI's and ACS's National Breast Cancer Awareness Month, drug maker Zeneca was given an endorsement by the NCI for its breast cancer prevention drug tamoxifen, while neglecting to inform women that its use significantly increases a woman's chance of developing uterine cancer. In a four-page press release regarding breast cancer, the NCI likewise failed to disclose to the public the significant association between certain chemicals and breast cancer. Zeneca is owned by Imperial Chemical Industries—the maker of several chemical carcinogens.[59]

- 1998: Former NCI Director Samuel Broder stated in an interview with the *Washington Post* that "the NCI has become what amounts to a government pharmaceutical company."[60]
- 2004: Nobel laureate and president of the Fred Hutchinson Cancer Control Center, Leland Hartwell, stated that the majority of the NCI's $4.7 billion budget is put toward "promoting ineffective drugs" for terminal diseases.[61]
- 2009: Doubts were cast on the impartiality and veracity of the material published in the *Journal of the National Cancer Institute* when researchers from the University of Michigan published a review of conflicts of interest in clinical cancer research. The review uncovered that the studies published in this and other journals were more likely to report higher patient survival rates if there were conflicts of interest reported.[62]
- 2010: In a letter sent to NCI director Dr. Harold Varmus U.S. Senator Chuck Grassley inquired about the several trips made by "numerous NCI employees, notably senior leadership," to international conferences that were bought and paid for by outside organizations or companies.[63]

A Cancer Industry Insider Speaks Out

In 1974, a young science writer named Ralph Moss began working at the world-renowned Memorial Sloan-Kettering Cancer Center (MSKCC) in New York. Just a few years later, at age thirty-four, Moss was promoted to the position of assistant director of public affairs. As part of his job, Moss drafted press releases and reported to the media on the latest developments in cancer research carried out at the hospital.

While composing the in-hospital newsletter one month, Moss was drawn to the research of Dr. Kanematsu Sugiura. In several experiments, Sugiura had shown that mice given a natural compound known as amygdalin (also known as laetrile, or vitamin B17) experienced a considerable reduction in tumor size.[64] Excited over the positive test results, Moss reported Dr. Sugiura's success to MSKCC's director of public affairs and other senior staff. In an article, Moss described the unexpected response of his superiors:

> They insisted that I stop working on this story immediately and never pick it up again. Why? They said that Dr. Sugiura's work was invalid and totally meaningless. But I had seen the results with my own eyes! And I knew Dr. Sugiura was a true scientist and an ethical person. Then my bosses gave me the order that I'll never forget: They told me to lie. Instead of the story I had been planning to write, they ordered me to write an article and press releases for all the major news stations emphatically stating that all amygdalin studies were negative and that the substance was worthless for cancer treatment. I protested and tried to reason with them, but it fell on deaf ears.[65]

Dumbfounded by the hospital staff's rejection of a promising natural cancer treatment, Moss set out to investigate why these individuals opposed releasing the study. He quickly discovered that the leadership at MSKCC had close ties to businesses that stood to lose millions if an effective, inexpensive, and nontoxic cancer treatment were readily available. Moss found that a high-ranking board member at the hospital was, in fact, the chairman of pharmaceutical company Bristol-Myers Squibb—at the time the world's largest manufacturer of chemotherapy drugs. His investigation revealed that seven of the nine people serving on MSKCC's powerful Institutional Policy Committee had conflicts of interest with the pharmaceutical industry, and that even the hospital itself had made investments with Big Pharma.[66] Moss brought to light that most of the members sitting on the hospital's board of directors were investors in petrochemicals and other industries manufacturing carcinogenic products. Tobacco companies Philip Morris and RJR Nabisco were also represented on the Board.[67]

Taking a big risk, Moss stood at a press conference in November 1977 and explained to the public how MSKCC had withheld the promising research on amygdalin as a tool against cancer. It was only one day later that Moss was fired from his position at the hospital. Shortly after his departure, I arranged for a meeting at my apartment between Moss and journalist Steve Dunleavy of the *New York Post*. As a result of this meeting, Moss' story received national attention when it was covered on the front page of the *New York Post*. Since his departure from the cancer establishment, Moss has gone on to be an outspoken proponent of numerous alternative cancer therapies and has written several books exposing the pervasive conflicts of interest that characterize the cancer industry.

Despite the work done by Moss and others to spotlight this issue, it has yet to receive sufficient media coverage. Meanwhile, the infiltration of MSKCC by special interests has continued. The late Richard Gelb, who served as the vice chairman of the MSKCC board, also worked as the CEO of Bristol-Myers Squibb.[68] The president and CEO of MSKCC from 1980 to 1999, Dr. Paul Marks, worked as director-emeritus of Pfizer and was employed as a consultant to Merck and other bio-pharmaceutical firms.[69] The current president of MSKCC, Dr. Craig B. Thompson, also sits on the board of directors for the pharmaceutical company Merck.[70]

In their servitude to special interests, our preeminent cancer research centers have poured their resources into ineffective projects while refusing to accept or even examine proven strategies of prevention and viable alternative treatments. While the work of MSKCC, the ACS, and the NCI has yielded little progress, these organizations continue to reap massive profits from the American people. We now take a deeper look into the issue of how our government fails to meaningfully address the enormous issue of daily exposure to carcinogens.

The Unregulated Poisons in Our Midst

Given their strong ties to big business, it is little wonder that the ACS and NCI resist acknowledging the dangerous carcinogens in our midst that, if made public, could threaten the profitability of the groups and their corporate affiliates Fortunately, not every one of our national cancer authorities is as beholden to special interests; the aforementioned President's Cancer Panel recently took a refreshingly honest look at the link between environmental pollutants and cancer. The panel's 2010 report discussed our national officials' denial of such a connection and stressed the need for expanded federal oversight of cancer-causing chemicals used in the manufacturing of plastics, moisturizers, sunscreens, and even food. The experts sitting on the committee urged President Obama to "use the power of your office to remove the carcinogens and other toxins from our food, water, and air that needlessly increase health care costs, cripple our nation's productivity, and devastate American lives."[71] The following pages describe some of these toxins, with particular focus on the causes and effects of our exposure to them.

Bisphenol-A (BPA)

Bisphenol-A, or BPA, is a plasticizer widely used to manufacture food and drink can linings, plastic bottles, cash register and credit card receipts, cosmetics and personal care products, dental sealants, microwave oven dishes, medical devices, and more. While useful as a chemical that promotes smoothness and ease of flow, bisphenol-A is an endocrine disrupter that imitates estrogen and can lead to debilitating or even fatal health conditions related to estrogen excess. The President's Cancer Panel noted that "more than 130 studies have linked BPA to breast cancer, obesity, and other disorders."[72] A 2007 review of approximately 700 studies on BPA published in the journal *Reproductive Toxicology* determined that children in utero and infants are especially vulnerable to the toxic hormonal effects of this substance.[73]

The response by regulatory agencies to the evidence of BPA's toxicity has been virtually nonexistent. In January 2010, the FDA quietly published an "update on BPA" which alluded to the potential danger of children being exposed to this ubiquitous chemical found in food packaging and plastic baby bottles. In reality, the agency has taken no regulatory action on this issue that has significant consequences for the health and livelihood of millions of Americans.[74] In the spring of 2012, after years of pressure the by food safety advocacy groups and a lawsuit brought against the FDA by the Natural Resources Defense Council, the agency was forced to make a decision on whether or not to institute a ban on the plasticizer. In an apparent effort to avoid press coverage, the FDA chose to announce late in the day on Friday, March 30, that they would not take action to remove BPA from food packaging.[75]

The BPA controversy has also touched the Susan G. Komen for the Cure foundation, which is the nation's foremost group whose stated mission is to fight breast cancer. The nonprofit recently came under fire for posting material on its website that denies a link between breast cancer and BPA. Bizarrely, the organization placed the claims while sponsoring research into the possibility of such a link.[76] The foundation's reluctance to admit such a correlation is far more explicable when investigating their major donors from the private sector. It turns out that Susan G. Komen for the Cure is financed by several corporations whose products contain BPA.[77] These sponsors include the Coca-Cola Bottling Company, General Mills, and Koch Industries.[78]

Formaldehyde

The President's Cancer Panel's report also discussed the lack of federal oversight and regulation for formaldehyde, a known carcinogen. Formaldehyde is commonly found in a broad range of consumer goods including clothing, mattresses, shampoos, nail polishes, and lotions, and is added to resins used in the manufacture of telephones and other molded appliances. Formaldehyde is present in almost all homes, as it is used extensively in plywood, foam insulation, carpeting, and other domestic materials. It is estimated that two million Americans are exposed daily to significant amounts of this substance while working.[79] Despite its association with nasal, breast, blood, and other cancers, the use of formaldehyde is neither regulated by our government nor required to be disclosed by manufacturers. It was not until 2011 that the Department of Health and Human Services' National Toxicology Program issued its Report on Carcinogens, which classified formaldehyde as a known human carcinogen. Incidentally, the release of the document was delayed for years while lobbyists from chemical trade groups such as the American Chemistry Council disputed the science behind the report.[80]

Foods that Kill

In 1995, the Cancer Prevention Coalition compiled a list of unlabeled and labeled toxins present in two foods regularly consumed by Americans: beef frankfurters and whole milk. While the notorious DDT has been phased out since that time, it is still found in animal products and human tissues. A growing list of studies has strongly linked frankfurters and milk with an array of ailments including colorectal, prostate, and breast cancers.[81, 82]

The list:

<u>Beef Frankfurters</u>—(e.g., Oscar Mayer Foods Corporation)

Unlabeled Toxic Ingredients

Benzene Hexachloride: Carcinogenic.
Dacthal: Carcinogenic (can be contaminated with dioxin); irritant; strong sensitizer.
Dieldrin: Carcinogenic; xenoestrogen.
DDT: Carcinogenic; xenoestrogen.
Heptachlor: Carcinogenic; neurotoxic; reproductive toxin; xenoestrogen.
Hexachlorobenzene: Carcinogenic; neurotoxic; teratogenic.
Lindane: Carcinogenic; neurotoxic; damage to blood-forming cells.
Hormones: Carcinogenic and feminizing.
Antibiotics: Some are carcinogenic, cause allergies and drug resistance.

Labeled Ingredient
Nitrites: Interact with meat amines to form carcinogenic nitrosamines, which are a major risk factor for childhood cancers.

<u>Whole Milk</u>—(e.g., Borden or Lucerne)

Unlabeled Toxic Ingredients

DDT: Carcinogenic; xenoestrogen.
Dieldrin: Carcinogenic; xenoestrogen.
Heptachlor: Carcinogenic; neurotoxic; reproductive toxin; xenoestrogen.

Hexachlorobenzene: Carcinogenic; neurotoxic; reproductive toxin.

Antibiotics: Some are carcinogenic, cause allergies and drug resistance.

Recombinant Bovine Growth Hormone (rBGH) and IGF-1: Risk factor for breast, colon, and prostate cancers.[83]

These foods are by no means exceptional. The scientific literature indicates that consuming staples of the Standard American Diet including processed foods, refined sugar, products with trans fats (partially hydrogenated oils), farmed fish, soft drinks, fried food products, and many other foods, significantly increases the risk of certain cancers (see part II).[84]

A report released by the National Cancer Institute in March 2011 revealed that childhood cancer rates shot up 9.4 percent between 1992 and 2007.[85] To account for this marked increase, some point to the increased use of toxic food additives and preservatives in recent years. The results of studies done by researchers at the United Kingdom's University of Southampton and the Center for Science in the Public Interest (CSPI) implicate common food additives and preservatives as entirely avoidable carcinogens. The CSPI's analysis found that several dyes, including the three most popularly used food dyes (Yellow 5, Yellow 6, and Red 40), were contaminated with known carcinogens.[86] These dyes are commonly added by major food producers to their products for purely aesthetic purposes. The dyes have no nutritional value yet can be found everywhere from Pillsbury Crescent Rolls to Kraft Barbecue Sauce, Doritos, Entenmann pastries, and a broad assortment of candies.

Danger Is More than Skin Deep

Much like the hazardous chemicals that contaminate our food supply, a wide range of dangerous compounds can be found in the majority of our cosmetic and personal care products. Despite the fact that the majority of these products contain cancer-promoting poisons, virtually every one of them is unregulated by the FDA. There are no safety reviews carried out for cosmetic and personal care products before they hit the shelves, and companies are not required to divulge any information about adverse events that may have occurred during internal trials. In a March 2011 article published in the journal *American Nurse Today*, Kate Bracy, MS, RN, NP, explains the FDA's inaction regarding this issue:

"The European Union (EU) banned certain phthalates known to cause reproductive defects after a 2002 study found phthalates in 80 percent of the products tested. The EU has now banned more than 1,000 chemicals from personal-care products. By comparison, the FDA has banned only 10. . . . The chemical industry has strenuously resisted these efforts by lobbying and filing lawsuits in states that attempt to pass protective bills."[87]

In the graph below, Bracy spotlights certain dangers present in everyday personal care products.

Toxins in personal-care products
This chart provides a partial list of toxins that may be found in some personal-care products, along with their possible effects.

Ingredient	Possible toxic effects	Where it's found
Acrylamide	• Cancer	• Conditioners • Moisturizers • Skin masks
Butylated hydroxyanisole (BHA), butylated hydroxytoluene (BHT)	• Cancer • Endocrine disruptions	• Conditioners • Blush • Eyeliners and eye shadows • Eyebrow pencils • Face powders, foundations • Lipsticks • Moisturizers
Dibutyl phthalate	• Birth defects • Fertility problems • Endocrine disruptions	• Fragrances • Nail polish

Ingredient	Possible toxic effects	Where it's found
Diethanolamine (DEA), triethanolamine (TEA)	• Cancer • Skin irritation	• Many personal-care products
Formaldehyde	• Cancer	• Nail polish
Lead acetate	• Reproductive or developmental toxicity • Possible carcinogenic effects	• Facial cleansers • Hair color and bleach • Lipstick
Mercury (thimerosol, indicated by ingredients starting with "mercur-")	• Reproductive or developmental toxicity • Possible carcinogenic effects	• Artificial tears • Eyedrops • Mascara • Pain or wound treatments
Parabens (methylparaben, butylparaben, propylparaben)	• Allergies • Endocrine disruptions	• Used as a preservative in many personal-care products
Talc	• Cancer if inhaled or used in genital area	• Baby powders • Bath powders • Deodorant • Solid makeup (blush, eye makeup)
Toluene	• Reproductive or developmental defects	• Nail polish

While the dangers associated with several cosmetic ingredients have been firmly established by science, a shocking 89 percent of all ingredients in personal care products have gone untested.[88] Laughably, the manufacturers of these products are responsible for policing their own goods.[89]

In 2010, the David Suzuki Foundation published a list of the "dirty dozen" chemicals added to cosmetics that damage the health of consumers. The chemicals listed that have been associated with increased cancer risk include the following:

- **BHA (butylated hydroxyanisole) and BHT (butylated hydroxytoluene):** Used as a preservative in lipsticks, moisturizers, and other products. Also used as preservative in foods such as cereals, butter, meats, and beer.
- **Coal tar dyes: P-phenylenediamine and colors listed as "CI" followed by a five-digit number or Blue 1:** A ubiquitous ingredient in cosmetic products, drugs, and foods.

- **DEA, cocamide DEA, and lauramide DEA:** Used widely in soaps, shampoos, and cleansers to make them foamy or adjust pH levels.
- **Paraben, methylparaben, butylparaben, and propylparaben:** Preservatives present in 75 to 90 percent of cosmetics.[90]

The scholarly research of the David Suzuki Foundation also proves that those personal care products that purport to be "natural" and nontoxic are often anything but. Discussing the incidence of contamination by 1,4 dioxane—a chemical that some studies have linked with cancer—the publication tells us that "in a study of personal care products marketed as 'natural' or 'organic' (uncertified), U.S. researchers found 1,4 dioxane as a contaminant in 46 of 100 products analyzed."[91]

While the flagrant lack of regulation of these chemicals may be confounding at first glance, the situation becomes much more understandable as we examine the collusive union between the corporations manufacturing these unsafe ingredients and the agency to which they should be answering—the FDA.

The FDA: (Not) Regulating for Special Interests

As one of the country's chief regulatory agencies, the U.S. Food and Drug Administration (FDA) is charged with ensuring the safety of our food, personal care products, and medical devices. But from its inception, the FDA's track record on health and safety has been nothing short of dismal. From allowing lethal drugs to be marketed and sold, to wasting tax dollars shutting down small businesses selling natural products such as raw milk and elderberry wine, the FDA displays the hallmarks of an enforcer for powerful corporate interests. A look into recent headlines provides more than enough evidence to support this claim.

Poison Poultry? OK with the FDA

In the summer of 2011, an FDA-commissioned study was released showing that an ingredient added to chicken feed known as

Roxarsone was contaminated with the potent carcinogen arsenic.[92] The results of the study forced the FDA to finally admit that cancer-promoting chemicals are present in animal feed. For years before this revelation, the FDA had made the erroneous claim that any arsenic in the diet of chickens was excreted through feces.[93] In reality, various levels of this harmful chemical appeared in the chicken meat sold in supermarkets across the United States and was consumed by many thousands of people. The news didn't come as a shock to many public health safety advocates who had long questioned use of Roxarsone–Maryland state legislators who worried that arsenic added to animal feed could make its way into the Chesapeake Bay had even acted to ban the substance.[94] The form of arsenic found in the feed was inorganic and even more noxious than naturally occurring organic arsenic.

The FDA never mandated the ingredients maker, Alpharma, to suspend sales of the carcinogenic feed, although the company opted voluntarily to do so.[95] The FDA even gave Alpharma thirty days to enact the suspension, assuring the public that "maintaining sales for this period will not pose a risk to human health"[96] And despite its admission of carcinogenic chicken meat after years of denial, the agency quickly issued a statement from Michael Taylor, the FDA's deputy commissioner for foods, attempting to deflect public disquiet by saying that the research raised "concerns of a very low but completely avoidable exposure to a carcinogen."[97]

As it happens, Taylor is far from trustworthy on issues of public health. His professional history is a perfect example of the FDA's dangerous subservience to the whims of powerful corporations. After spending seven years lobbying on behalf of genetically modified (GMO) food pioneer Monsanto, Taylor became a policy chief at the FDA, where he spearheaded the effort to legalize Monsanto's genetically engineered recombinant bovine growth hormone (rBGH) in spite of evidence of its deleterious health effects.[98]

Furthermore, Alpharma is a subsidiary to drug giant Pfizer—a large client of the FDA that pays millions of dollars to the agency to review its pharmaceuticals.[99] Similar to the personnel at other pharmaceutical firms and corporations, Pfizer retirees often go on to work at the FDA as consultants or administrators, and vice versa.[100] This revolving-door scenario ensures that the interests of Big Pharma are well represented in an agency that claims to be an impartial arbiter of American health and safety.

It should be pointed out that arsenic-based drugs are still used today in the feed of turkeys and pigs, and we are only beginning to see their full effects. It has made national news recently that most of our domestic rice supply is now contaminated with arsenic because of its presence in the animal food industry. Officials are now struggling to claim that arsenic occurs naturally in rice despite the fact that rice has been arsenic-free for thousands of years. This problem has led pediatricians to warn parents against feeding their infants rice cereal or rice milk, while South Korea has suspended its purchases of rice from the United States.

The FDA's current Code of Federal Regulations provides guidelines for Nitarsone, a pharmaceutical fed to turkeys that contains arsenic. According to the regulations, turkeys that don't have a sufficient water supply while consuming the feed may experience leg weakness or paralysis.[101] The regulations also advise turkey farmers to "discontinue use five days before slaughtering animals for human consumption to allow elimination of the drug from edible tissues."[102] While the FDA considers this questionable animal feed entirely acceptable for turkeys bred for human consumption, the agency explicitly states that "the drug is dangerous for ducks, geese, and dogs."[103] Given the FDA's track record in this arena, it is reasonable to question Nitarsone's potential threat to public health.

Seafood that Sickens

The catastrophic offshore oil spill of 2010 poured nearly five million barrels of oil into the Gulf of Mexico. Among the far-reaching consequences of this environmental disaster were the widespread destruction of marine life and the contamination of major United States fisheries by chemical toxicants. Health safety advocates raised their concerns that seafood coming from the Gulf might contain high levels of cancer-causing polycyclic aromatic hydrocarbons (PAHs) resulting from the oil plume. In response to these worries, the FDA formulated a set of guidelines known as levels of concern (LOCs) for PAHs in seafood produced by these fisheries.

In a study published in the journal *Environmental Health Perspectives* titled "Seafood Contamination after the BP Gulf Oil Spill and Risks to Vulnerable Populations: A Critique of the FDA Risk Assessment," a research team at the Natural Resources Defense Council (NRDC) set out with the objective of evaluating the "degree to which the FDA's risk criteria adequately protect vulnerable Gulf Coast populations from cancer risk associated with PAHs in seafood."[104] The vulnerable populations examined in the study included pregnant women, children in utero, and people who consume above-average amounts of seafood. In addition to their scientific analysis, the research team—which was led by Miriam Rotkin-Ellman—pored over internal FDA documents obtained through the Freedom of Information Act (FOIA).

The study found that the agency's shoddy risk assessment of PAHs exposed Americans to seafood contaminated with levels of carcinogens between 100 and 10,000 times what is recognized as safe.[105] The authors determined that 2 out of every 100 pregnant women who consumed quantities of shellfish deemed acceptable by the FDA would give birth to children who were at a significant risk of developing cancer.[106] While probing internal agency documents, the team uncovered email messages in which employees at the FDA and EPA expressed doubts over the standards set forth in the agency's risk assessment criteria. The NRDC team also found unreleased assessments of the contamination. Such revelations are compelling evidence of widespread and deliberate deceit regarding Gulf seafood's lethal toxicity.

FDA personnel publicly rejected the NRDC study as too conservative, but provided no evidence to support their claim. In an interview with Alternet, Rotkin-Ellman countered the FDA's criticism, saying that such baseless declarations beg "the question of whether or not it was a political versus a scientific decision."[107]

In point of fact, Rotkin-Ellman's assertion is well founded; the FDA is lobbied every year by hundreds of special interests looking to sway federal policy. Given the FDA's dangerous lack of regulation in the case Gulf seafood, it should come as no surprise that the agency was lobbied in 2010 by organizations with a huge stake in seafood sales. These organizations include the Catfish Farmers of America, the Southern Shrimp Alliance, and the National Fisheries Institute, which represents the entire industry.[108] The American Chemistry Council—the same organization that fought to prevent the government's acknowledgment of carcinogens in health care products—was one of the top groups to lobby the FDA that same year.

These facts elucidate one critical point: The FDA would rather appease the purveyors of toxic foods and other products than institute measures that could prevent millions of Americans from being exposed to deadly carcinogens. We see again how the extensive control of special interests has put us at a greater risk of developing cancer and other conditions. The next section of this book will uncover deeper fraud and deception as we probe the disturbing politics of cancer care.

Mainstream Prevention and Detection—More Harm than Good?

Reevaluating the Conventional Approach

Not only does modern medicine irresponsibly emphasize cancer treatment over prevention but many of the prevention methods pushed on patients by the medical-industrial complex are highly questionable. It turns out that some of the most popular techniques in use today are often unsuccessful and dangerous. While the inadequacies of conventional preventive medicine result in undue harm to millions of patients, there are several parties that profit tremendously. These include biotechnology, pharmaceutical, and insurance firms as well as hospitals and clinical laboratories.

Mammography Mendacity

We have a health care system in the United States that emphasizes early diagnosis and treatment. On face value this seems like a logical and prudent approach. However, testing healthy individuals for microscopic signs of illness places a strain on time, money, and resources, while the tests themselves can be invasive, harmful, and even fatal. There is perhaps no better example of this than the $5 billion[109] American women spend annually on mammograms. Lauded as a tool that saves lives, mammograms have become more controversial in recent years as a host of critics and consumers have begun to take a deeper look into the science behind this popular test. A mammogram is an expensive exam that requires a slew of health care professionals: a skilled technician to do the procedure, one or two board-certified radiologists to interpret the results, and a primary care physician to discuss the results. A suspicious finding usually requires a repeat mammogram, possibly a surgeon, a surgery suite, a nurse, an anesthesiologist to do a biopsy, a pathologist to interpret those results, and a return to the primary care physician. How many thousands of dollars does this add up to so far? And how much stress and anxiety does it create for the woman who worries about the outcome? Studies show that women may experience severe psychological distress for up to a year or more as a result of a breast cancer scare.[110]

Nowhere in this scenario are women warned about the dangers of mammograms. Despite races for the cure and other relentless paid advocacy programs compelling women to undergo this painful procedure, mammograms are still a crude and inaccurate diagnostic test for breast cancer. There are large numbers of both false positives and false negatives, meaning that women will be told they have cancer when they don't, and told they don't have cancer when they do. A large Swedish study concluded that an incredible 70 to 80 percent of all women with a positive mammographic diagnosis of cancer were found not to have cancer on biopsy.[111] Over the course of the next decade, American women are expected to spend as much as $70 billion on unnecessary surgeries stemming from false positive mammogram results.[112]

It is estimated that for 2,000 women who receive mammograms regularly over a ten-year period, one life will be saved, but ten more will undergo needless and harmful treatment for cancer that they don't have—including chemotherapy, radiation, and even breast removal.[113] Conversely, a supposed clean bill of health from a normal mammogram result is not something that should cause any woman to breathe a sigh of relief. Many women have a negative mammogram only to discover a suspicious lump on their own a few weeks or months later. It is estimated that a full 40 percent of women between ages forty and forty-nine will have breast cancer that goes undetected by mammography.

Far worse than the fact that mammograms do not provide reliable results is the dangerous levels of ionizing radiation emitted by the diagnostic device itself. According to Dr. Samuel Epstein, the amount of radiation from a mammogram is 200 times that from a chest X-ray. Meanwhile, research presented at the Radiological Society of North America's 95th Scientific Assembly and Annual Meeting in 2009 incriminated low-dose radiation as a key factor in the development of breast cancer. The research demonstrated that women were 2.5 times more likely to develop breast cancer if they had received either a mammogram or chest X-ray before the age of twenty.

The cancer industry tells us that more women have breast cancer than ever before, but the survival rate has increased because of mammograms and early treatment. We are not made aware that a significant percentage of the increase in breast cancer is due to mammograms finding cancer that isn't there, which possibly explains the improved cure rate. Nor are we made aware that the definition of breast cancer has changed significantly since the advent of mammograms. A frequently overlooked statistic shows that the rate of one type of breast cancer, ductal carcinoma in situ (DCIS), has skyrocketed by 328 percent since mammograms were first introduced in the 1970s.[114] DCIS is a condition that can only be found by mammography, because these lesions are too small to be picked up by physical examination. DCIS is currently the most common diagnosis resulting from breast tissue biopsy, but is DCIS even breast cancer at all? Ductal carcinoma in situ is actually a *precursor lesion* for breast cancer. Rather than cancer itself, a precursor lesion is a collection of cells that could grow into breast cancer, but also might not—we simply cannot know and have no way to predict the outcome. DCIS has been called the poster child for uncertainty, as it remains unclear whether the condition poses a serious threat to women's health. Studies of DCIS that were missed at biopsy suggest that the lifetime risk of progression to cancer if untreated is very low.[115]

The mammography industry is very powerful and has worked successfully to prevent other means of breast cancer identification from being developed. In fact, studies show that thermography, an increasingly popular test that is noninvasive and does not emit radiation, may be more effective at identifying breast cancer than conventional mammography. While a mammogram begins to detect cancer clumps of about four billion cells, thermographic imaging may be far more sensitive, picking up abnormal growth as small as 256 cells.[116] However, we must keep in mind that so-called "early detection" is a dangerously misleading term because finding cells that are a variation from normal is not the same thing as identifying cancer. There are many abnormal cells that never progress to malignancy, and we truly cannot tell the difference in most cases. Thermograms, like mammograms, hold the potential for disease mongering by finding abnormal cells that will not develop into cancer, thus bringing women into a destructive treatment regimen for which they have no need.

There is an enormous conflict of interest between our cancer authorities and the promoters of mammography—no fewer than five American Cancer Society presidents have been radiologists specializing in mammography. In light of such industry influence, it should come as no surprise that the ACS has consistently adopted policies favorable to the companies that make mammogram machines, such as DuPont, Siemens, and General Electric. DuPont, in fact, was a major sponsor for the group's ACS Breast Health Awareness Program, an initiative that encouraged women to receive mammography screenings while failing to publicize the scientifically established methods of prevention that would help them avoid the disease altogether.[117] Another disturbing conflict of interest lies in the fact that the ACS actually contracts with the mammography industry to conduct cancer research,[118] which calls into question the impartiality of such research.

A series of well-funded campaigns have prompted women to undergo regular mammograms, which are promoted as safe, responsible, and necessary. But as the Cochrane Review has concluded in their meta-analyses from both 2001 and 2011, the currently available reliable evidence does *not* show a survival benefit of mass screening for breast cancer. A Canadian study published in *The Lancet* went further, stating that "since the benefit achieved is marginal, the harm caused is substantial, and the costs incurred are enormous, we suggest that public funding for breast cancer screening in any age group is not justifiable." Despite all this, the NCI continues to recommend that all women should submit to mammograms every two years beginning at age forty. Our current promotion of "breast cancer awareness" leading to widespread mammography is simply drawing more healthy women into the patient pool rather than saving lives. Women would be better served by learning what they can do to improve their chances of never developing breast cancer. This includes eating a healthy, plant-based diet free from processed foods and animal products, exercising, losing weight, and avoiding environmental toxins that are known to cause breast cancer.

The Trouble with Biopsies

Most of us never give a second thought to biopsies. We consider them routine and harmless when, in fact, biopsies have been shown to pose considerable risk to patients. For example, studies by researchers in North America, Europe, and Asia indicate that the risk for developing serious infection from prostate cancer biopsies could run as high as 5 percent.[119] Because the prostate gland is buried amidst the intestines, the ultrasound-guided needle used in the procedure has the potential to transport antibiotic-resistant bacteria from the bowel into the prostate, bladder, or bloodstream. One Canadian study concluded that out of 10,000 men given a prostate biopsy, 9 died within a month from infections.[120] Another study published in the *Journal of Urology* last year indicated that 7 percent of all men aged sixty-five and older are hospitalized within thirty days of having a prostate biopsy. In contrast, men in the same age bracket who have not been given a prostate exam were half as likely to end up in the hospital.[121] These statistics are especially alarming given the popularity of this test, which is administered to more than one million American men each year. More disconcerting is that mainstream physicians are required to administer a biopsy to make an official diagnosis of cancer.

Infection is not the only risk attached to needle biopsies. Even more concerning is the fact that sticking a needle into a tumor can cause seeding of cancer through the entire trajectory of the needle, spreading it farther and more quickly than if left untouched. A study done by a team of researchers from John Wayne Cancer Institute in California showed that, for patients with cancer, a biopsy done with a fine- or large-gauge needle may actually increase the spread of tumor growth by up to 50 percent compared to the rate of metastasis for patients who are given more traditional excisional biopsies, or lumpectomies. Other evidence now suggests that men receiving prostate exams are just as likely to die from prostate cancer as those who do not submit to exams. A study published In 2011 in the *British Medical Journal* that analyzed the prostate cancer mortality rate of 1,494 men over the course of twenty years, found that the "rate of death from prostate cancer did not differ significantly" between those men who were screened and those in the control group.[122] This report came on the heels of a 2009 investigation published in *The New England Journal of Medicine* in which researchers discovered that only one out of every 1,400 men given prostate screenings would have their life saved by early detection.[123] Moreover, the study's authors noted that out of the pool of 1,400, nearly 50 of the men would end up being treated for cancer unnecessarily.[124]

The results of a recent study on the genetics of malignant tumors has prompted many in mainstream medicine to question the usefulness of biopsies in the fight against cancer. Published in *The New England Journal of Medicine* in 2012, the study concluded what alternative health practitioners have long known—that genetic mutations can vary greatly throughout a cancerous growth.[125] The findings reveal that biopsies, which probe only a small part of the overall mass, are not always indicative of the overall genetic activity. Alarmingly, many doctors formulate treatment plans and select drugs for their patients based on a single biopsy.

Colonoscopies Reconsidered

Once considered a foolproof screening tool for potential colon cancer, colonoscopy has shown itself to be a possibly dangerous and unnecessary procedure. Routine colonoscopy is often recommended once every ten years starting at age fifty, with the purpose of finding polyps in the colon before they become cancerous.[126] However, the polyps removed via colonoscopy are mostly adenomatous[127]— meaning slightly abnormal, but not cancerous—with no certainty of ever developing into cancer.[128]

Meanwhile, the colonoscopy procedure can be hazardous. A semi-flexible colonoscope must travel through six feet of convoluted bowel loops,[129] making four right-angle turns along the way.[130] The procedure is not always problem-free, with serious complications occurring in 5 per 1,000 U.S. cases.[131]

Serious risks associated with colonoscopy include internal bleeding, complications from sedatives[132] and perforation of the intestine which can lead to disability or death.[133] Additionally, excessive stress and permanent damage to the kidneys can occur as a result of improper hydration during the three day bowel cleansing regimen prior to the procedure.[134]

The risks involved with colonoscopy have led the U.S. Preventative Services Task Force to advise against regular colonoscopies for people ages seventy-six to eighty-five, saying that the procedure's risks outweigh its benefits for individuals over eighty-five.[135] Researchers at Yale University Medical School determined that colon cancer tests on certain populations of ill patients may often do more harm than good.[136]

Despite these observations, costly overuse of colon cancer screenings is widespread amongst Medicare patients. While the $2,000 operation is recommended every ten years, a study published in *Archives of Internal Medicine* revealed that nearly half of the Medicare patients reviewed had undergone a repeat exam less than seven years after receiving normal results.[137] Research suggests that hospitals, health care practitioners, and biotech firms make untold millions each year while foisting unnecessary risk on seniors.

Conventional Treatments: Big Money, Small Results

The Procrit Model

Recent revelations regarding Procrit, a popular anti-anemia drug manufactured by Johnson & Johnson subsidiary Ortho Biotech, bring the depraved machinations of the cancer industry into clear focus. In her 2011 book *Blood Feud: The Man Who Blew the Whistle on One of the Deadliest Prescription Drugs Ever*, Kathleen Sharp unearths the details of a campaign by Johnson & Johnson drug representatives to encourage prominent oncologists to prescribe more and more Procrit to their cancer patients with anemia. Sharp recounts one instance in which Dean McClellan, one of the company's foremost drug reps, "wined and dined" cancer doctors and their wives over the course of a weekend in a high-end California hotel. In *Blood Feud*, McClellan recalls that the goal of the meeting was to convince doctors to increase their prescriptions of Procrit to their patients from 30,000 units to 40,000 units per week.[138] Two things, however, stood in the way of his objective: The FDA had approved a maximum of 30,000 units for the medication, and federal regulations prohibited pharmaceutical firms to advertise anything beyond the approved dosage. Nevertheless, McClellan had a plan up his sleeve. Sharp explains what happened next:

> So, McClellan, a star rep and medical consigliere, led a "discussion" about high-dose experiments. Taking his cue, one physician explained how he routinely injected patients with 40,000 units of Procrit. Another oncologist pumped his people with 10,000 units for ten consecutive days—triple the approved amount. "That seems a little extreme," said McClellan, frowning.
>
> "Oh no," the doctor said. "I haven't seen any side effects so far."
>
> A few months later, Procrit sales hit the $1 billion mark, beating Amgen by a hair. The resort trip had certainly helped. But it was just one part of an expansive, long-running off-label marketing campaign, according to sales documents. Slowly but surely, oncologists around the country began administering so many high Procrit doses that, in time, the off-label therapy became the "community standard."[139]

While Johnson & Johnson's devious marketing scheme is outrageous in and of itself, even more troubling is the fact that Procrit has been shown for years to be a dangerous medication which, while able to correct anemia, has the unfortunate tendency to cause sudden death.[140] Confronted with proof of its extreme toxicity, in June 2011 the FDA urged physicians to consider prescribing Procrit only to those individuals with severe anemia.[141] Federal regulators noted that the use of Procrit, along with other anti-anemia drugs Epogen and Aranesp, has been linked to an increased risk of heart attack and stroke and may even promote the spread of cancer.[142] The author of one of these studies, Dr. Anthony Reiman of the University of Alberta, Canada, stated in an interview that "the use of drugs to encourage red blood cell formation in cancer patients with anemia increases the risk of death and serious adverse events such as blood clots." Reiman added, "At best, these drugs don't seem to improve longevity."[143]

The controversy over Procrit provides us with an excellent example of how the medical mafia promotes ineffective cancer treatments just to turn a profit while disregarding the negative side effects. The extent of the death and damage caused by this toxic medication will never be known, but one thing is for certain: American taxpayers have spent more than $60 billion on this drug for Medicare patients alone since it hit the market in 1989.[144] In this next section, we will see that the deception perpetrated by the medical-industrial complex goes much deeper than just one medication.

The common approach to cancer utilizes three main therapies: chemotherapy, radiation, and surgery. A deeper look into each of these approaches reveals them to be potentially harmful and largely ineffective in the long term. Why does the medical establishment promote these treatments regardless of their poor track record on safety and efficacy? For the answer, we simply have to follow the money trail. Today, the average total cost of medical care for cancer patients, from diagnosis to death, is $350,000.[145] In some cases the cost can exceed $1 million.[146] There is no doubt that cancer is Big Business, and our costly overreliance on current treatment methods is the result of a coterie of special interests conspiring to capitalize on human suffering.

Chemotherapy

The term "chemotherapy" refers to cancer treatment that uses strong drugs to inhibit cell growth and division. These drugs may be administered orally or intravenously, usually as part of a cyclical regimen. According to the American Cancer Society, chemotherapy drugs may be used to

- Keep the cancer from spreading
- Slow the cancer's growth

- Kill cancer cells that may have spread to other parts of the body
- Relieve symptoms such as pain or blockages caused by cancer
- Cure cancer[147]

While chemotherapy manages to kill some cancer cells, a large body of research shows that the majority of patients undergoing this treatment will benefit only slightly, if at all. Chemotherapy does not kill all of the cancer cells in a person's body, nor does it prevent eventual regrowth of these cells. Moreover, the side effects of chemotherapy are often devastating and can actually promote cancer growth, including the new growth of a completely different type of cancer. By all indications, it is time to carry out a critical reassessment of this popular therapy.

Chemotherapy came into existence in the mid-20th century when Dr. Cornelius P. Rhoads explored the potential therapeutic use of mustard gas used during WWI in curbing cancer. Rhoads based his studies on the observations of Dr. Louis Goodman and Dr. Alfred Gilman, whose research demonstrated that the blood of soldiers exposed to nitrogen mustard during warfare had abnormally low levels of white blood cells. Because the gas was observed to retard the division of somatic cells, the researchers postulated that this toxic spray used in warfare could also be used to slow the multiplication of cancer cells. Chemotherapeutic treatment was standardized in the 1950s and has been a fixture in the mainstream treatment of cancer ever since. Rhoads, who would later become head of the Memorial Sloan-Kettering Cancer Center, was one of chemotherapy's foremost proponents.

In his book *Questioning Chemotherapy*, Dr. Ralph Moss states that only 2 to 4 percent of all forms of cancer are effectively treated by chemotherapy.[148] Moss writes that in the other 96 to 98 percent of cancers, chemotherapy fails to eradicate the disease completely.[149] A 2004 study by researchers from the Department of Radiation Oncology at the Northern Sydney Cancer Centre in Australia discovered that chemotherapy treatment contributed to the five-year survival of a mere 2.1 percent of all patients in the United States.[150] One of the major reasons that chemotherapy fails to eliminate tumors is that cancer cells have the unique ability to quickly adapt in a toxic environment in order to survive. As a result, cancer cells can mutate and become resistant to chemotherapy drugs that target a specific type of cancer cell. Despite the documented ineffectiveness of chemotherapy, the vast majority of patients are not aware of this fact. Doctors rarely share this information with patients, and statistics representing the success of chemotherapy are routinely manipulated by the medical establishment to give the appearance that it works well.[151]

Chemotherapy causes a host of acute and sometimes lethal side effects. The treatment not only eliminates cancer cells but also kills healthy, normal cells. Such cytotoxicity leads to conditions including nausea, hair loss, anemia, permanent damage to the brain, heart, and liver, and death. The immunosuppressive effects of this treatment are significant and leave the body weakened and more vulnerable to infection and scores of other illnesses. In 2008, the United Kingdom's National Confidential Enquiry into Patient Outcome and Death (NCEPOD) reported that the use of chemotherapy caused potentially lethal side effects in four out of ten patients who received the drugs toward the end of life.[152] In addition, the report ascertained that chemotherapy hastened the death of 27 percent of all patients who were given treatment thirty days before death.[153]

Lesser known side effects of chemotherapy may be equally harmful. A 2007 study published in the *International Journal of Gynecological Cancer* showed that tamoxifen, a chemotherapy drug used to prevent breast cancer in women, is associated with higher rates of uterine cancer incidence and mortality.[154] Some newer drugs, such as Avastin, work by blocking the blood supply to cancer cells. But these drugs may also block the blood supply to the GI tract, resulting in perforation and fatal bleeding. Another study published in 2010 by Danish researchers indicated that the toxicity of chemotherapy extends to oncology nurses. The study, which examined the health records of 92,000 nurses, discovered that individuals administering and handling such chemicals were more likely to develop breast, thyroid, nervous-system, and other cancers.

The financial burden of these treatments in considerable. The price of oral chemotherapy drugs, such as Avastin, Herceptin, and Tarceva, is astronomical, as the cost of some pills exceeds $90,000 a year.[156, 157] When patients are insured, monthly copays are typically around $1,000.[158] Provenge, a prostate cancer medication approved by the FDA in 2010, is a prime example of the obscene costs associated with modern cancer treatment. Prescribed only to men with "incurable" prostate malignancies, Provenge costs an astounding $93,000 a year. Much of the cost of this medication falls on taxpayers paying into Medicare, and, in other cases, the uninsured are forced to shell out exorbitant sums for a drug with very little ostensible benefit; the medication has been shown to extend the life of patients by just four months.[159]

It is critical to note that the four-month survival figure was taken from a study funded by the drug's maker, Dendreon. Furthermore, the study concluded that Provenge had no apparent effect on the progression of cancer. Such contradictory findings led the authors of another editorial published in the *New England Journal of Medicine* to question the validity of the study's conclusions.[160] More evidence of the systemic corruption surrounding cancer drugs came in early 2012, when Dendreon CEO Mitchell Gold stepped down from his position after accusations of fraud and misleading investors regarding the anticipated success of Provenge.[161]

Despite the evidence of chemotherapy's dangers and ineffectiveness, cancer patients are commonly led to undergo the treatment. The aforementioned NCEPOD report called attention to the fact that the use of chemotherapy was "inappropriate" in almost one-fifth of all cases reviewed.[162] Over the last few years, an increasing number of physicians and hospitals have revived a particularly devastating form of chemotherapy—"hot chemotherapy." The procedure combines invasive surgery with doses of heated chemotherapeutic agents poured directly into the abdominal cavity. Due to its questionable efficacy and gruesome side effects—which include death from infection and irrevocable damage to the body tissue—hot chemotherapy has been used traditionally to treat only rare forms of appendix cancer. Despite this, more physicians have begun utilizing hot chemotherapy—which can cost more than $100,000 per treatment—to treat common forms of colorectal and ovarian cancer.[163] Commenting on the growing popularity of the therapy, Dr. David P. Ryan, the clinical director of Massachusetts General Hospital Cancer Center, stated, "We're practicing this technique that has almost no basis in science."[164]

Surgery

For hundreds of years, surgery was the only method used to treat cancer. The use of surgery today has been grandfathered in and has little to do with randomized, double-blind clinical trials—modern medicine's standard measures of safety and efficacy.[165] While the surgical removal of cancerous tumors is vital to patient recovery in many cases, it is imperative to shed light on the harmful disadvantages of surgery on cancer patients.

The removal of a malignant tumor through surgery can effectively stimulate cancer growth. Removing a primary tumor from the body significantly reduces the amount of two proteins known as endostatin and angiostatin from the tumor site. These proteins help regulate the growth of tumor blood vessels, and once they are diminished, metastasis can proceed at a greatly accelerated rate. This problem is compounded by the fact that surgery suppresses the immune system by inhibiting the activity of the critically important cancer-fighting natural killer cells. Not only does this inhibition promote metastasis; it can also leave patients more susceptible to infection. Compromising immunity further still are the analgesic pain medications that are commonly given to patients after surgery. Analgesic drugs such as morphine inhibit natural killer cells, which are particularly important during recovery.

A study by researchers at Memorial Sloan-Kettering Cancer Center from 2009 showed the potentially lethal consequences of what many consider to be a routine surgical cancer treatment. The study, published in the journal *Cell*, examined the phenomenon known as self-seeding, in which cancer cells separate from a primary tumor and are transported to other parts of the body, only to return to the original tumor location, where they re-seed themselves.[166] Through this process, chemical reactions from the immune system can trigger stray cancer cells not removed during surgery to return to where they originated, promoting the growth of another tumor. The study's findings confirm that surgery, like chemotherapy and radiation, is often neither effective nor safe, as it fails to address the root causes of cancer from a holistic standpoint.

Given the various limitations of surgery and the abundance of effective natural approaches to fighting cancer, it would seem logical to minimize the number of costly surgeries. We find, however, that mainstream medicine readily promotes surgery even when the operation is likely to be risky, unsuccessful, or unnecessary. Dr. Laurence E. McCahill, of the Lacks Cancer Center in Grand Rapids, Michigan, found that almost half of all women who undergo breast cancer lumpectomy surgeries are unnecessarily subjected to a follow-up operation. McCahill's analysis showed that nearly half of the 2,026 women whose medical records were reviewed were operated on despite having test results showing no stray cancer cells—an indication that a follow-up surgery was likely of no benefit to the patient.[167]

A study published in 2011 in *Archives of Surgery* reviewing the outcomes of breast cancer surgeries for women in California showed that more than one-third of all mastectomies carried out were unnecessary. The findings showed that in 35.1 percent of all cases reviewed, the lymph nodes removed during the operation were not infected with cancer. Further still, the authors found that women with lower incomes were even more likely to undergo this disfiguring and invasive surgery needlessly.[168]

The Journal of the American Medical Association published a study that same year demonstrating that the common practice of removing malignant lymph nodes from the armpit offered no improvement in survival rates or relapse prevention.[169] The study concluded that one out of every five women had their lymph nodes removed unnecessarily.[170] Because removing these lymph nodes damages the entire lymphatic drainage system of the arm, this surgery can result in painful cellulitis and swelling of the arms to twice their normal size. Extrapolating the data, it stands to reason that each year, 40,000 women in the United States are put under the knife unnecessarily, risking complications such as serious infection and lymphedema.

Radiation Therapy

About one-half of all cancer patients being treated with conventional medicine will undergo some form of radiation therapy, often in combination with surgery or chemotherapy. The goal of radiotherapy is to damage the DNA in tumors by sending beams of ionizing radiation to the tumor in order to control and halt cancer cell growth. Despite its popularity as a treatment in the fight against cancer, the clinical evidence demonstrates that, in most cases, this approach to healing is not particularly safe or effective.

Much like surgery, radiotherapy was adopted as a standard practice after crude experimentation over a century ago that never proved its safety and efficacy. One of the chief pioneers in using radiation to treat cancer was the Polish-born Marie Curie. In her studies, Curie observed that inserting pellets of radium and polonium into tumors could cause them to shrink in size. Unaware of the dangers of highly radioactive materials, Curie's years of experimentation caused her to become very ill and succumb to aplastic anemia, a condition where the bone marrow stops producing red blood cells. Even today her notebooks are so highly contaminated by radioactivity that researchers are required to sign a waiver form in order to view them. Over the years, mainstream medicine has refined the radiotherapy techniques developed by Curie but the fact remains that in every case, this form of treatment exposes patients to harmful and sometimes lethal doses of radiation.

Radiotherapy causes numerous crippling side effects, including severe swelling, joint pain, fibrosis, dysphasia, infertility, stroke, and brain damage. Perhaps the ultimate irony of this form of treatment is that exposure to ionizing radiation in order to treat cancer is itself extremely carcinogenic. This is because radiotherapy not only damages the genetic material stored in cancer cells but also mutates genes in viable, healthy cells, increasing the likelihood they will later turn into cancer cells. In his book *World Without Cancer,* Edward G. Griffin writes that even though radiation manages to decrease tumor size in certain cancers, it is largely ineffective in eliminating neoplastic cancer cells, which are the true target of the treatment. Hence, radiation can often actually increase the malignancy of the tumor it is meant to control.[171]

Through statistical manipulation, the medical establishment distorts the efficacy of radiation therapy. For example, deaths from acute complications resulting from radiotherapy such as radiation necrosis are not labeled as cancer deaths, but cases in which the patient was "cured" by radiation.[172] This same misleading formula is applied when patients die from other conditions that are linked to radiation therapy, including stroke and heart disease.[173] Another deceptive tactic frequently used is claiming that patients who don't experience cancer growth within five years are fully recovered, even if the same cancer returns later on.[174]

A study out of the H. Lee Moffitt Cancer and Research Institute in Tampa, Florida, showed that women receiving radiation therapy for cancer of the left breast were more at risk of experiencing cardiovascular events such as heart attack. The study found that even ten to twenty years after being exposed to radiotherapy, women were 25 percent more likely to have coronary heart disease.[175] Another study conducted by researchers at Emory University and published in *Archives of Internal Medicine* revealed that individuals who submitted to radiation therapy as children were significantly more at risk for developing diabetes. Children who were exposed to total body radiation were discovered to be 7.2 times as likely to develop diabetes as those who did not receive radiotherapy.[176] One of the authors of the study noted, "As a result of their curative therapies, childhood cancer survivors face an increased risk of morbidity and mortality."[177]

Despite improvements over the years, newer radiation therapy technologies have been shown to damage patient health as well. A recent article written by the vice chairman of the Department of Urology and Chief of Robotics and Minimally Invasive Surgery at New York's Mount Sinai School of Medicine, David B. Samadi, M.D., pointed out the substantial dangers that accompany newer radiotherapy techniques practiced today. The article discusses the flaws of increasingly common treatments, such as stereotactic "radiosurgery" (also known as Cyberknife) and external beam radiotherapy, both of which involve directing a narrow beam of radiation at tumors through linear accelerator technology. Samadi explains that these blasts of radiation can result in serious damage to surrounding tissues because of excessive amounts of radiation being delivered or via defects in linear accelerators that cause the radiation to be "leaked," or directed into healthy body tissue.

These mistakes can lead to a multitude of complications, including difficulty speaking and walking, as well as ulcers, sores, and even untreatable holes in body tissue.[178] Layers of skin can die and slough off, leaving painful, ulcerated areas open to further trauma and infection. Irradiation of oral tumors can cause destruction of the soft tissues holding the teeth in place, causing them to fall out. These forms of radiation therapy have also been reported to induce comas and even cause death.[179] It is likely that many of these destructive complications go unreported, because the damage may take several months after treatment to manifest. A report by the *New York Times* detailed the heartbreaking case of Alexandra Jn-Charles, a thirty-two-year-old woman with breast cancer who was given doses of radiotherapy through a malfunctioning linear accelerator at three times the prescribed amount for the entire twenty-seven days of her treatment, without anyone noticing the error. The pain she suffered after the excessive radiation burned an actual hole in her chest was so excruciating that she, a mother of two young children, reportedly contemplated suicide.[180] But a short time later, Ms. Charles's radiation-induced injuries claimed her life.

An article written by German researchers in the journal *Cancer* in 2010 highlighted the sad reality of how patients are encouraged by the medical establishment to submit to damaging and ineffective radiation treatments during their final days. Despite claims that radiation can ease pain in terminally ill patients, the analysis showed that palliative radiation conferred no benefit to the majority of patients.[181] Worse still, more than half the individuals receiving radiotherapy experienced more pain and suffering as a result of the treatment, and 60 percent of the patients died while being treated.[182] In their conclusion, the authors of the study commented that such insistence on the part of doctors to extend radiation treatments unnecessarily was evidence of "overly optimistic prognoses and unrealistic concerns about late radiation damage."[183]

Investigating the economics of radiotherapy helps explain why such a barbaric treatment is possible in today's medicine. The answer, as always, is money. Radiation therapy is very profitable, despite the extra expenses for equipment, technicians, and the disposal of hazardous waste. Yet there are clear indications that many health care professionals and hospitals look for ways to drive up the price of radiotherapy to make the treatment even more financially rewarding. A study published in the *Journal of the National Cancer Institute* in 2011 concluded that the cost of intensity-modulated radiation therapy for women with breast cancer was five times higher in areas where Medicare paid for the procedure.[184] In an editorial that was published along with the study, doctors Lisa A. Kachnic and Simon N. Powell of Boston University Medical Center stated that the findings "would appear to confirm the suspicion . . . that medical decision making is too heavily influenced by reimbursement rather than medical necessity."[185]

Another analysis appearing the *Journal of Clinical Oncology* explored treatment costs of surgery and radiation for prostate cancer patients covered by Medicare. Evaluating a pool of 71,000 men between 2002 and 2005 and monitoring their progress through the end of 2007, the authors found a sharp rise in the use of more expensive treatments, such as intensity-modulated radiation therapy (IMRT).[186] Importantly, the more costly treatments examined in the study have never been proven to be any more effective than the less expensive alternatives examined by the team. The researchers commented that compared to the less costly alternative, the nationwide excess direct spending for the rapid adoption of more expensive therapies was $282 million for IMRT, $59 million for brachytherapy plus IMRT, and $4 million for MIRP for men diagnosed in 2005.[187] In other words, taxpayers spent an additional $345 million for more expensive cancer therapies that had never been proven to be any more effective than cheaper treatments.

Our medical system's reliance on toxic and damaging cancer treatments that regularly fail to cure or help patients crystallizes one key point: The largest beneficiaries of conventional cancer therapies are, unfortunately, not the patients themselves but the physicians, hospitals, biotechnology and pharmaceutical firms, and other groups that comprise the medical-industrial complex. The unadulterated scientific evidence and statistics documenting the poor outcomes of cancer treatment should make us stop and seriously question the widespread application of chemotherapy, surgery, and radiotherapy. Even more reason to reconsider their use is the well-documented success of many alternative approaches to cancer (see part II). Next, we will shift our focus from how the cancer industry readily endorses risky therapies that come with a big price tag to its brutal campaign to suppress effective and nontoxic natural cancer treatments that are inexpensive by comparison.

Fighting against a Cure: Suppressing Therapies that Work

Decades of Stonewalling Medical Brilliance

An investigation of our medical authorities' position on natural cancer therapies turns up extensive evidence of a determined effort to stamp out any cheap and efficacious therapy that could threaten the establishment's profitability. In my 1979 article "The Great Cancer Fraud" I explained how mainstream medicine seeks to marginalize practitioners of alternative medicine, even when they are highly esteemed scientists:

> Patrick McGrady, Sr., science editor for the American Cancer Society for twenty-five years before he resigned in disgust at the extent of its ineptitude, said that ACS officials "close the door on innovative ideas." A notable example is Dr. Linus Pauling, who has come up with some very positive findings to show that vitamin C can extend cancer survival manyfold. This eminent scientist, who is the only living person to have won the Nobel Prize twice, never had any trouble getting grants before he became

involved with vitamin C. Since then he has been rejected by the American Cancer Society as well as by the National Cancer Institute research grant committees five times.[188]

More than thirty years later, we find that nothing has changed: The cancer establishment employs a range of dishonest and sometimes sinister tactics to ensure that the profits continue to flow. A prime example of the backlash faced by individuals who use effective holistic cancer treatments is Dr. Max Gerson.

Dr. Max Gerson

In "The Great Cancer Fraud," I documented the hardships faced by Dr. Max Gerson in promoting his alternative cancer therapies. Dr. Gerson was a German physician who in the 1920s was able to cure his own migraine headaches through diet after conventional remedies failed him. He later adapted this same diet, which was salt-free and vegetarian, to treat and cure lupus and tuberculosis. While he meticulously documented his research and published scientific papers in several issues of *Medizinische Welt*, the concept that disease could be cured through diet invited ridicule. Eventually Dr. Gerson left Germany for the United States. He settled in New York City in 1936, where he opened a clinic and successfully cured patients of cancer with his controversial diet. What follows are excerpts from my article:

> Max Gerson was repeatedly attacked, most violently by his own colleagues, and his New York clinic fought to survive for many years. Cancer patients came to Gerson as a last resort. When—in many cases—they became cancer-free, their former doctors sometimes destroyed records confirming that they even had the disease
>
> In 1946 the U.S. Senate invited Gerson to hearings on a bill to authorize funds for research on the prevention and cure for cancer. He appeared and presented five cancer-free patients and

their case histories before a Senate committee, all members of which were impressed with his findings. The favorable, 227-page Congressional Committee Report—document #89471—now gathers dust in the archives of the Government Printing Office. A newspaper reporter who inquired was informed that there were "no copies left." Just five years after the congressional hearings, Gerson was not allowed to practice at any New York hospital and found it difficult to secure assistants. Up until then he had, for over twenty years, demonstrated excellent results in treating cancer. His approach was on a highly scientific level, and his credentials were the finest. Yet Gerson never received a penny from cancer-funding agencies to aid his research. He was the victim of a by-now-familiar cancer blackout: The inventor is isolated; the medical journals won't publish his work; and when he publishes elsewhere, they say it is "not scientific."

Meanwhile, the graves were filling up with the frightening and awful mutilations of operating and X-ray rooms: those burned and butchered victims turned out of hospitals to go limping hopelessly toward their final rest, those poisoned victims of toxic chemotherapy whose every body cell had tasted the painful effects of a full-scale chemical assault. "Nothing more could be done for them," said the medical establishment. They had already had their checkups, sent in their checks, and traveled the same worn, one-way road to suffering and death.[189]

Despite that many thousands of cancer patients have experienced a rapid recovery following the Gerson protocols, this therapy remains unendorsed by the medical establishment and is even claimed to be "dangerous" by groups such as the ACS.[190] Dr. Gerson's daughter, Charlotte Gerson, continues her father's work through the two Gerson clinics—one in Mexico and the other in Hungary—where hundreds of patients are helped to heal from cancer and other diseases each year (see part II).

Dr. Lawrence Burton

An exposé of the cancer industry that I wrote with Leonard Steinman in 1980 was titled "The Politics of Cancer: Suppression of the New Cancer Therapies: Dr. Lawrence Burton."In the article, I discuss how Dr. Burton's effective early detection system for cancer as well as promising cancer treatments were suppressed by the forces behind orthodox medicine.[191] Burton invented a treatment known as immuno-augmentative therapy (IAT), which involves injecting cancer patients with naturally occurring blood protein mixtures designed to bolster the body's immunity.

In my investigative report thirty-four years ago, I wrote about the harassment of Burton at the hands of groups such as the NCI and ACS. The NCI, along with the Memorial Sloan-Kettering Cancer Center, first tried to buy out Burton by offering to give him and his colleagues a paltry one-year $15,000 research grant in exchange for exclusive control over the therapy that was built on years of diligent research.[192] When Burton refused to accept such terms, he quickly became the target of ridicule by the medical establishment. In a classic Catch-22 scenario, all of Burton's requests to publish his research in medical journals were refused, while his petitions for funding by the NCI were denied on the grounds that his research had not been published.[193]

Confronted with such staunch institutional opposition in his own country, Burton moved his clinical practice to the Bahamas. After being pressured by the NCI and other American health authorities, the Bahamian government shut down Burton's practice in 1985, claiming that patients who received care at the clinic could have been exposed to injections contaminated with the AIDS virus. In the aftermath, it was clear that the decision to close the clinic had much more to do with Burton's establishment-threatening therapy than a public health issue.[194] It turned out that thousands of blood samples collected from clinics across the United States had tested positive for the AIDS virus, yet Burton's operation was the only one forced to close.[195] Dr. Harold Jaffe, then serving as director of the Center for Disease Control's AIDS program, admitted that the laboratory tests officials used to check for contamination of the clinic's materials were highly inaccurate and often produced false positives.[196] Further, Jaffe commented that more reliable tests were available.[197] In 1986, Burton was allowed to reopen his practice in the Bahamas.

In my article, I made a prediction about the future of Burton and his treatment:

> Despite the fact that no one has disproved Burton's theories, he remains on the American Cancer Society's blacklist. As long as his work is maligned by the ACS as "unproven," he will continue to be thought of as a quack, a charlatan, a fraud, by country-club doctors more concerned about maintaining the medical status quo than about actively seeking the relief of human suffering.[198]

And so it remained until Burton passed away thirteen years later in 1993 after having enjoyed considerable success in treating more than 4,500 cancer patients at his clinic in Freeport.[199]

The groundless blackballing of great scientific minds like Pauling, Gerson, and Burton are far from exceptional. Today, Stanislaw Burzynski, M.D., Ph.D., of the Texas-based Burzynski Clinic, stands at the center of such egregious mistreatment by mainstream medicine.

The Burzynski Saga

Dr. Burzynski has become well known over the last thirty-five years for devising safe and effective anticancer therapies involving the peptides and amino acid derivatives known as *antineoplastons* (see part II). His work, however, has been highly disrupted by the medical establishment.

I was one of the first journalists to report on Burzynski's groundbreaking medical innovation and the resistance to it by our health officials when I published an article in *Penthouse* in 1979 titled "The Suppression of Cancer Cures." Just a few years into his work treating cancer patients with this very promising and nontoxic technique, Burzynski was being denied research funds by the NCI and ACS and became the target of attacks by mainstream medicine.[200] While his experiments and procedures followed established protocols for safety and transparency, Dr. Burzynski was put under investigation by his local medical society with no explanation of their motives or reasoning. Today, Dr. Burzynski continues to face systematic blacklisting from the medical establishment.

One of the primary institutions to challenge Burzynski has been the FDA. Despite repeated petitions to the FDA for a review and approval of his antineoplaston treatments, the agency spent decades groundlessly denying a proper review of Burzynski's work and depriving the public of a proven tool in the fight against cancer. In an effort to revoke his medical license, the FDA pressured the Texas medical board in the 1980s to charge Burzynski with violating a law that did not exist.[201] Representatives of the Texas board of medical examiners went so far as to track down patients who had been treated by Burzynski and attempted to convince them to take legal action against their former doctor.[202]

The FDA convened no fewer than five grand juries in the 1980s and 1990s in their attempts to indict Dr. Burzynski on claims of wrongdoing. More disgraceful still are the huge sums paid out by the American people to finance the government's dubious charges; for the second grand jury alone, $60 million was allocated to fund the investigation.[203] Incidentally, the first four grand juries failed to result in an indictment, while two trials stemming from the fifth investigation found Burzynski not guilty on all charges. After nearly twenty years, the FDA finally gave in to pressure from the public and members of Congress, authorizing Burzynski to carry out clinical trials of antineoplaston therapy in 1996.[204] This did not stop the FDA from concurrently moving forward with their legal battles against the physician and his clinic. In an article appearing in the *Washington Post* that year, it was written that "the prosecution marks the first time the FDA has tried to jail a scientist for using a drug on which he is conducting FDA-authorized clinical trials."[205]

After begrudgingly accepting to conduct research on Burzynski's antineoplaston therapy in the late 1990s, the NCI followed in the footsteps of the FDA and did its best to suppress the treatment. To begin, the NCI prematurely closed the trials before they were completed.[206] Scientists conducting the study failed to administer any antineoplastons to seven out of the nine patients enrolled in the trials, while the other two patients were given dosages far below the recommended amounts.[207]

The recently released film *Burzynski: The Movie*, directed by Eric Mercola, further exposes the federal government's campaign to silence this doctor and discredit his contributions to medicine. It is a must-see for anyone looking to better understand categorical corruption within the world of cancer. In April 2012, the trial of the *Texas Medical Board v. Stanislaw Burzynski* was set to begin after two years of intense litigation. A week before the trial, however, most of the charges against Burzynski were dropped by the administrative law judges, leading the board ultimately to move to dismiss the case, which was officially dismissed November 12, 2012.

Blocked by Big Medicine

Numerous pioneers of promising natural and nontoxic cancer therapies have been victimized by the medical establishment. What follows are some of the most remarkable examples of how such medical tyranny operates:

- Despite having outstanding success using alternative therapies to help patients overcome cancer, Dr. Nicholas Gonzalez found it impossible to have any of his findings published in any reputable scientific journal during the 1990s. When his therapy was finally given the opportunity to prove itself in NCI-sponsored clinical trials, they were sabotaged by obviously biased overseers.[208]

- After having outstanding success treating seriously ill cancer patients with his immunotherapy techniques, German physician Josef Issels was the target of attacks by the German government as well as groups such as the ACS. Even though there existed several scientific studies attesting to the efficacy of Issels' therapy, he was entirely written off by the ACS as a practitioner of "unproven methods" and never given the chance to have his practice observed.[209]

- Seemingly threatened by the promise of Royal R. Rife's energy-based cancer therapy he developed in the 1930s, Morris Fishbein of the American Medical Association (AMA) went about intimidating physicians who were using the Rife technology and brought a court case against Rife.[210]

- Dr. William Koch, the inventor of an oxygen-based cancer treatment known as glyoxylide, was persecuted by the AMA and FDA throughout his career. He was brought to trial twice by the FDA but was never convicted. Barry Lynes reported in *The Healing of Cancer: The Cures, the Cover-Ups and the Solution Now* that Koch had at least thirteen unsuccessful attempts on his life during his career.[211]

- Harry Hoxsey, the man behind the herbal anticancer treatment known as Hoxsey Therapy (see part II), spent decades defending attacks from mainstream medicine against his successful and nontoxic approach to cancer. From the 1920s onward, physicians who worked with Hoxsey's cancer patients were stripped of their licenses, and clinics practicing the therapy were forced to close through heavy-handed intimidation by Morris Fishbein and the AMA as well as the NCI.[212] So intense was the persecution Hoxsey faced in the United States that he relocated his practice to Tijuana, Mexico.[213]

Conclusion

For nearly a century, the innovators and practitioners of holistic cancer treatments have been unfairly maligned and attacked by the medical establishment. In case after case, it is clear that the cancer industry seeks to marginalize these individuals and their proven therapies in order to preserve the status quo—an immensely lucrative system that promotes and profits from human suffering. If the natural and effective approaches to cancer treatment in existence today were finally embraced by the mainstream, the foundation of the medical paradigm——based on rampant greed and dishonesty—would quickly collapse. The dedication of Stanislaw Burzynski, Nicholas Gonzalez, the Gerson family, and many others to pursuing holistic cancer treatments in the face of such hostility has laid the foundation for a new paradigm that is gaining momentum.

Shifting the Medical Paradigm

More and more people are waking up to the corruption that plagues our medical system and choosing to seek out alternatives to conventional medicine, especially when it comes to cancer treatment. The credibility of our medical officials diminishes with each passing day as proof of their extensive conflicts of interest and moral degeneracy continues to make headlines. Today more than ever, a diverse collection of physicians, nurses, activists, and health advocacy organizations are standing up to the medical-industrial complex and calling for fundamental changes to the way health care is managed in this country. Their efforts are helping curb the rampant medical fascism that leaves millions of Americans penniless, maimed, or dead. Nevertheless, to be victorious in the war on cancer and the larger war for health freedom, we must challenge the flawed dogmas that guide modern medicine, and we must demand accountability from our government health officials and their industry overlords for choosing revenues over the health and safety of the American people every step of the way. This crooked racket has caused enough unnecessary suffering; it's time to take our health back into our own hands.

PART II

A NATURAL APPROACH TO CANCER PREVENTION AND TREATMENT

Cancer Defined

Cancer is a group of diseases in which abnormal cells, instead of being killed by the body's immune system, multiply and spread. The cells no longer follow the rules for the usual orderly progression of growth and become renegades. Cancer can attack any part of the body and may spread to other parts. The sites most often affected are the skin, the digestive organs, the lungs, the prostate gland, and the female breasts.

Before exploring what happens in cancer, let's look at the life cycle of a healthy cell. A healthy cell starts out as immature and then goes through routine changes to mature. As a mature cell it performs whatever job in the body it is supposed to do, and then it gets old and dies. Along the way, the active mature cell needs maintenance. There are genes in the cell that do the job of repairing mistakes and keeping the cell in running order.

Cancer occurs when the cell doesn't mature, doesn't repair its mistakes, or doesn't die. There are two types of cancer: those that form tumors and those that don't. When these outlaw cancer cells are regular building-block cells, like cells in the breast, lung, prostate, or skin, tumors occur. These cancers show up as abnormal masses or tumors because the cells are replicating out of control, heaping up into big masses, and killing the normal cells around them.

Cancers can also be in non-building-block cells. This type of cancer doesn't produce a tumor and occurs in the cells of the blood. The blood cells go out of control, resulting in cancers like leukemia and lymphomas. These blood cells remain immature. They proliferate and push out and kill the regular healthy mature blood cells. They show up in the bone marrow or clog up the lymph nodes or the spleen.

Then there is a really tricky part of cancer, and the part that can lead to death, which is when the aberrant cells migrate. They metastasize and invade other parts of the body, setting up shop in parts of the body distant from their original site. For instance, prostate cancer likes to invade the bones and brain. Breast cancer cells like the bones and the liver. The cancer cells develop the ability to spread by making special enzymes that cut through cell walls and travel through the blood.

What makes the cell go haywire? No one can answer for sure. But what can we do to prevent cancer? What can we do to fight cancer once the cells have gone out of control? There is a lot to say in response to these questions. First, poisonous elements from the environment can cause the cell to become cancerous, things like asbestos and cigarettes (see part I). But it also turns out that some people are more inclined to get cancer than others are. Genetic predisposition and environmental assaults appear to provide the powerful one-two punch.

Early Warning Signs

Among the early warning signs of cancer are a change in bowel or bladder habits; unusual bleeding or discharge; a thickening or lump in the breast, testicles, or elsewhere; an obvious change in a wart or mole; a persistent cough or hoarseness of the voice; a sore throat that does not go away; and difficulty swallowing or indigestion.

Conventional Treatment

In conventional medicine, the usual treatment for cancer is surgery to remove the tumor, radiation to blast away tumors, and/or administration of powerful drugs that find and kill the cancer cells. Unfortunately, these treatments are very difficult to endure and don't always work (see part I). Surgery leads to disfigurement. Radiation can cause fibrosis (scarring) and eventually infertility, joint issues and secondary cancer. Chemotherapy essentially poisons the body in order to kill the tumor. It is toxic because it introduces a poison into the body, and it is invasive because the poison aggressively invades the cells and tissues of the body. The problem is that the poison is indiscriminate. It kills not only cancerous cells but healthy ones as well. In fact, its invasion of the body is systemic (total), not local, and therefore seriously damages the immune system. Chemotherapy drugs are very toxic to healthy cells and can make you feel really sick—your hair falls out, you can't eat, you're weak, and you're deeply fatigued.

Alternative Approaches

Another approach is to try to get the body itself to fight the cancer. Remember that a normal cell has its own maintenance team that repairs damage. If that part of the cell can be bolstered and reactivated, it can do its job of overcoming the tumor-forming oncogenes, reactivating the cell's tumor suppressor genes, and subduing the cancer's growth. Whenever this has occurred, the cancer goes into remission and disappears. Taking care of yourself and living a healthy lifestyle is the best way to start.

So what can each of us do to prevent cancer? Engaging in regular physical activity is essential. Volumes of research have established that regular exercise supports the immune system and promotes psychological well-being, which is also critically important. It's been theorized that people who tend to suppress anger are more prone to cancer than are others, and that people who are happier and more content with their lives tend to have less cancer and fight it more successfully. It is important to learn to release emotions in a constructive way so as not to be overwhelmed by them, and this entails addressing one's own personal needs, as opposed to living according to other people's expectations. Among those practices found to benefit cancer patients' mental welfare are hypnosis, breathing exercises, massage, aromatherapy, yoga, and positive visualization.[214]

Of course, for the prevention and treatment of cancer, it is critical to use common sense. The number-one killer of all types of cancer is lung cancer, so you should avoid tobacco at all costs. And because being overweight or obese is especially harmful to the body and the immune system, it is critical to maintain a normal weight.

DIET

Although generally dismissed by the medical establishment as irrelevant, diet and nutritional factors are among the most important contributors to cancer development. Because so many chronic diseases, including cancer, are related to eating a diet poor in phytonutrients, fiber, vitamins, and minerals but rich in fat, processed ingredients, and additives, it is of paramount importance to consider the importance of adopting a highly nutritious, plant-based diet. Cancer has been linked to diets that are high in fats, animal products—even certain types of vegetable proteins—and processed foods. Pesticides and some types of food additives also can cause cancer. But just as diet can harm you, it can also prevent cancer. What follows is a comprehensive list of anticancer foods.

Alkaline Foods

The vast majority of Americans consume an excess of acid-forming foods. Research has shown that tumor growth increases in an acid environment.[215, 216, 217] The blood is maintained in the body at a slightly alkaline level of between 7.2 and 7.4. Eating alkaline foods keeps the blood pH in its ideal range, which is important for the prevention and treatment of cancer. Ideally, the diet should consist of 80 percent alkaline-forming foods, such as those available from many raw fruits and vegetables, as well as nuts, seeds, grains, and legumes. What follows is a list of recommended alkaline-forming foods:

Fruits: Berries, apples, apricots, avocados, bananas, currants, dates, figs, grapefruit, grapes, kiwis, lemons, limes, mangos, melons, nectarines, olives, oranges, papayas, peaches, pears, persimmons, pineapple, quince, raisins, raspberries, strawberries, tangerines, and watermelon. (The most alkaline-forming foods are lemons and melons.)

Vegetables: Artichoke, asparagus, sprouts, beets, bell peppers, broccoli, Brussels sprouts, cabbage, carrots, cauliflower, celery, collards, corn, cucumbers, eggplant, endive, ginger, horseradish, kale, kelp, seaweeds, mustard greens, okra, onions, parsley, potatoes, radishes, spinach, squash, tomatoes, watercress, and yams.

Whole Grains: Amaranth, barley, oats, quinoa, and wild rice.

Beans/Legumes: Almonds, chestnuts, chickpeas, green beans, lima beans, peas, and soybeans.

Seeds: Alfalfa, chia, coconut, radish, and sesame.

In addition balancing the body's pH through a mostly alkaline diet, the following foods stand out as beneficial in preventing and treating cancer:

Cruciferous Vegetables

Vegetables in the cruciferous family include kale, cabbage, broccoli, cauliflower, arugula, watercress, turnips, mustard plant, Brussels sprouts, and bok choy. Cruciferous vegetables contain detoxifying compounds called indoles and isothiocyanates, which have been proven to help prevent and reverse cancer.[218, 219, 220, 221] Recent research has identified sulforaphane, a compound found in broccoli, cabbage, and other cruciferous vegetables as a potent anticancer agent.[222] Packed with raw and all-natural kale, broccoli, Brussels sprouts, and other cruciferous vegetables, cruciferous vegetable powders are a rich source of anticancer nutrition.

Green Foods

Wheatgrass, barley grass, alfalfa, blue-green algae, arugula, spinach, chlorella and spirulina, and other green foods are rich in blood-purifying chlorophyll and other important phytonutrients for detoxifying the system and rejuvenating organs. Laboratory tests have established that chlorophyll inhibits the activity of carcinogens at a molecular level.[223] Studies have demonstrated the capacity of chlorophyll-rich foods to reduce tumor growth.[224, 225, 226] Containing spinach, chlorella, spirulina, barley grass juice powder, and fifteen other detoxifying vegetables, certain green powders are loaded with phytonutrients proven to be highly beneficial in cancer prevention and healing.

Red Foods

Research confirms that red foods such as strawberries, tomatoes, raspberries, tart cherries, cranberries, and goji berries are high in immunosupportive and cancer-fighting nutrients such as lycopene and carotene.[227, 228, 229] Many red foods also have high antioxidant content, making them an integral component of any anticancer diet. The antioxidant power of raspberries, strawberries, pomegranate, and dozens of other nutrient-rich fruits make some red and berry powders cancer superfoods.

Fiber

Though not a food itself, fiber is an important component of fruits, vegetables, and whole grains. The typical American diet includes about 14 g of fiber each day, which falls short of what is necessary for cancer prevention. Studies have indicated that 30g of dietary fiber daily decreases the risk of colorectal cancer. Research has also suggested that high fiber intake may lower the risk of breast, colorectal, uterine and prostate cancers.[230, 231, 232]

Olive Oil

Olive oil has been shown to possess anticancer properties. Studies have demonstrated that the monounsaturated fatty acids contained in olive oil have a protective effect against cancer growth.[233, 234] Research has also shown that the phytochemicals abundant in olive oil inhibit cancer growth in vitro.[235] But remember, more isn't always better. Olive oil still has 120 calories per tablespoon, so don't go overboard. For maximum benefit, olive oil should be used in moderation. Choose a good-quality, extra virgin, cold-pressed variety.

Juices

Freshly squeezed fruit and vegetable juices provide valuable enzymes and antioxidant nutrients that are easily digestible. Compounds in cabbage juice have been observed to have favorable effects on stomach and colorectal cancer.[236, 237] Rich in beta-carotene and vitamin A, carrot juice is beneficial but should be watered down, as it is also high in sugar, and can potentially spike blood sugar levels.[238] Adding a teaspoon of vitamin C to juices creates an even more potent preventive tonic.

Green Tea

High in antioxidants known as polyphenolic catechins, green tea has been shown to help prevent skin, lung, esophageal, stomach, pancreatic, and bladder cancer in animals.[239] Studies have demonstrated that green tea extract halts the spread of chronic lymphocytic leukemia.[240] Recent research also indicates that green tea contains compounds that considerably slow the growth of cancer cells.[241]

Mushrooms

Several varieties of mushrooms have powerful healing properties. The maitake mushroom kills cancer cells by enhancing the activity of T-helper cells.[242] Research has shown the maitake mushroom to exert a favorable effect on various types of cancer, including breast, colon, and prostate.[243, 244, 245] Both shiitake and reishi mushrooms have also been observed to have strong antitumor properties in animals.[246, 247, 248] Research has revealed that the cordyceps mushroom inhibits the division and proliferation of cancer cells.[249] And, surprisingly, the common white button mushroom has been shown to suppress aromatase activity and estrogen biosynthesis, which make it an excellent breast cancer chemopreventive agent.[250]

Macrobiotic Foods

Proponents of macrobiotic eating claim that cancer patients following this approach lead longer and better-quality lives. In several cases, cancer patients deemed incurable by mainstream medicine have reported full recoveries on a macrobiotic diet. Success may be due to high levels of antioxidant nutrients and a low amount of fat. In fact, the total percentage of calories from fat in macrobiotic diets is approximately 10 to 12 percent, a 30 percent drop from the average American diet. Best results with the macrobiotic diet are seen with endocrine-related cancers, such as cancer of the breast, prostate, pancreas, uterus and ovaries. This is because with these cancers, too many fat cells produce or synthesize estrogen and androgen hormones that contribute to the disease; reducing the amount of dietary fat lessens hormone production.

Seaweeds

Chinese medicine has long recognized the value of seaweed for treating cancers, as it softens hardened tumors. More recently, research has shed light on the powerful mix of micronutrients, including Vitamin C and Vitamin E, as well as minerals, iodine, fiber, and polysaccharides in seaweed, which make it a powerful nutritional tool in combating cancer.[251, 252] Considered to be one of the healthiest populations on earth, the Japanese consume more seaweed than any other nation.

Spices

Spices offer numerous health-promoting benefits, and certain spices have been found to aid in the prevention and treatment of cancer. Research has associated black pepper and cumin intake with a lower incidence of colon cancer.[253, 254, 255] Rosemary is known to help prevent DNA damage by carcinogens and suppress cancer cell proliferation.[256, 257, 258] Capsaicin, an ingredient found in chili peppers, kills prostate cancer cells.[259] Evidence suggests that parsley combats lung and breast cancer.[260, 261]

ANTIOXIDANT SUPPLEMENTS

The value of antioxidants, particularly beta-carotene; vitamins A, C, and E; flavonoids; selenium; glutathione; superoxide dismutase; and coenzyme Q10 cannot be overestimated in disease fighting and prevention. Antioxidants attack free radicals before they do irrevocable damage. Many clinical studies confirm their protective effects, while other research shows that antioxidants increase a patient's tolerance of chemotherapy and radiation.

Vitamin C

Vitamin C is the prime nutrient when it comes to overall support of the immune system. When fighting cancer, large quantities are required both orally and intravenously. For decades studies have established the importance of vitamin C intake in preventing and reversing breast, gastric, ovarian, and many other forms of cancer. [262, 263, 264, 265, 266] Orally, bowel-tolerance levels are recommended; that is, one should take an amount that almost causes diarrhea. (Most people can tolerate up to 12 g daily of vitamin C, dividing this dose throughout the day.) But for best results, intravenous vitamin C drips are needed as well. Research indicates that this method supplies the greatest healing effects because more of the vitamin can be easily tolerated. Patients are often given between 50 and 100 g of intravenous vitamin C, which is an excellent jump-start to any health protocol. This treatment relieves pain and nausea, often making painkilling drugs unnecessary. High doses of intravenous vitamins C and A are associated with long-term survival of a variety of cancers, even after they have metastasized. Despite claims that vitamin C may disrupt chemotherapy treatments, recent studies have established that vitamin C kills tumor cells without interfering with the effectiveness of chemotherapy.[267, 268]

Alpha-Lipoic Acid

This is a powerful antioxidant that neutralizes the hydroxyl radical (which plays a role in all stages of cancer growth) as well as other free radicals. It boosts glutathione, which combats the damaging cytokines, and regenerates vitamins C and E and coenzyme Q10. Further, alpha-lipoic acid has been shown to activate the anticancer caspase enzyme, induce cancer cell apoptosis, and suppress metastasis.[269, 270, 271] The recommended dose is 250 to 500 mg per day. One can take 500 mg three times daily at maximum.

Essential Fatty Acids (EFAs)

Omega-3 fatty acids block important causes of cancer. Omega-3 fatty acids can suppress dangerous cytokines, as well as the stress-induced pro-inflammatory cytokines IL-6 and IL-10. While some fish oils are a rich source of Omega-3s and have been found to reduce the risk of skin, breast, and prostate cancer,[272, 273, 274] not all fish have a good Omega-3/Omega 6 ratio, and it is important to know where fish came from and to avoid farmed fish at all costs. Remember, fish don't synthesize Omega-3 fatty acids on their own; they obtain it from eating green vegetable matter. So boosting your intake of green leafy vegetables with high Omega-3 contents will also provide high dietary levels of this valuable antioxidant. The suggested doses of the fatty acids are 1,000 mg of perilla oil, which provides 550 to 620 mg of linoleic acid; 1,000 mg of flaxseed oil, which is rich in omega-3 fatty acid, seven times per day; and four capsules of the formula MegaEPA (available from Life Extension), which contains 2,400 mg of EPA/DHA. Cancer patients can take up to eight to twelve softgels per day combined with four Mega GLA softgels.

Vitamin A

Vitamin A reduces infections and tumors, and is especially noteworthy for its ability to clear the lungs of smoke and other pollutants.[275, 276, 277] Studies of animals show a definitive link between vitamin A deficiency and higher cancer risk.[278, 279] Emulsified vitamin A comes from fish oil and is easy to digest. Vitamin A also comes from non-animal sources, such as lemongrass, wheatgrass, and carrots. Because vitamin A is fat-soluble and not excreted by the body, excessive intake can be dangerous, inducing hypervitaminosis A, which causes cells to swell and rupture, leading especially to central nervous system toxicity. But large quantities of vitamin A are needed for this to happen, and it is safe at the recommended dosage. Four thousand to 7,000 IU of vitamin A, from supplemental and food sources, are recommended daily—less if beta-carotene is taken.

Beta-Carotene

The liver converts beta-carotene to vitamin A as needed, making it a safe source of the vitamin, especially for women of childbearing years, as no fetal problems are associated with it. (Note: People with liver problems may be unable to convert beta-carotene into vitamin A.) In addition, beta-carotene itself stimulates T-helper cells, which prevent the development of cancer. Further studies have demonstrated beta-carotene protects against lung and colon cancer. Fifty thousand international units taken daily may prevent cancer in cigarette smokers. For general purposes 20,000 to 30,000 IU of beta-carotene is extremely helpful.

Carotenoids

Carotenoids are the naturally occurring pigments found in various plants. With oncology, mixed carotenoids are important as free radical scavengers.[280, 281] Lycopene is associated with low risk of breast, prostate, lung, and colon cancers.[282] There is an inverse relationship between beta-carotene and thyroid carcinoma. Lutein offers protection against breast cancer in premenopausal women.[283, 284] Suggested doses are 9 to 20 mg of sulforaphane, 10 to 30 mg of lycopene, and 15 to 40 mg of lutein, along with a mixed carotenoid blend containing alpha- and beta-carotene.

Flavonoids

Bright colors in fresh fruits and vegetables are usually indicative of flavonoids, which are phytochemicals that are efficient free radical scavengers. Citrin, hesperidin, quercetin, and rutin are names of some of these disease-fighting substances. Studies suggest that flavonoids help prevent damage to DNA, neutralize carcinogens, and lower the risk of lung cancer.[285, 286, 287]

Vitamin E

Much like vitamin C, vitamin E prevents cancer by preventing free radical damage, and activating immune system cells against tumors and infections.[288, 289] In clinical studies, 400 to 1,200 IU daily have been shown to help patients with breast or cervical cancer.[290] Vitamin E works especially well when taken in conjunction with 200 mcg of selenium.

Vitamin K

Mounting evidences points to vitamin K, a potent antioxidant with anti-inflammatory properties, as a powerful tool in the prevention and treatment of cancer. Abundant in leafy greens, vitamin K has been shown to inhibit the progression of liver cancers and shows great promise for treating numerous types of cancer, including prostate and lung cancer.[291, 292, 293] The recommended dose of vitamin K is 2,100 mcg daily.

Selenium

This trace element, which is involved in DNA metabolism and the health of all cell membranes, has antioxidant properties, promotes apoptosis (cancer cell destruction), acts as an immunological response modifier, and plays a part in cancer prevention and treatment.[294,295,296] Supplementation of selenium can improve the quality of life during aggressive cancer therapies. The suggested dose is 200 mcg per day; the optimal dose could range from 200 to 400 mcg daily.

Silibinin (Milk Thistle)

The major active constituent of milk thistle is a long-recognized antioxidant that has recently discovered anticarcinogenic qualities.[297,298,299] Milk thistle is an adaptogenic herb. It produces repair where it's needed or shuts down cell production in tumor cells. Silibinin encourages differentiation in malignant cells, blocks the activity of the enzyme COX-2, and, by cutting off the vascular network of the tumor, inhibits the growth of drug-resistant breast and ovarian cancer lines. The recommended dose of milk thistle is 100 mg twice daily.

Glutathione Peroxidase

Glutathione is found in every cell of our bodies, where it plays a major role in defending our systems. Studies show that low levels of glutathione increase the risk of cancer, AIDS, and chronic fatigue syndrome.[300] To stimulate glutathione production, L-glutathione and N-acetyl-cysteine (NAC, a precursor of glutathione) should be taken.

Superoxide Dismutase and Catalase

Much like glutathione, these antioxidants are frontline defenses against free radical damage, and are especially protective of the heart, brain, lungs, kidney, and liver.

Coenzyme Q10

Coenzyme Q10 works in conjunction with other enzymes in the body to optimize energy. Specifically, Q10 improves oxygen utilization, acts as a stimulus to the immune system, and serves as an antioxidant, all of which are important in cancer prevention and treatment.[301, 302] Studies have made the connection between Q10 deficiency and increased risk of breast cancer and melanoma.[303] A dose of 500 mg daily is recommended for cancer patients.

Grape Seed Extract

Grape seeds contain pycnogenol, a powerful disease-fighting antioxidant. Pycnogenol, among its various age-retardant abilities, slows cell mutations. Intake of grape seed extract has been linked with significant decreases in the risk of developing colon, prostate, and breast cancers.[304, 305, 306, 307] The suggested dose is 200 to 500 mg daily.

Dimethyl Sulfoxide (DMSO)

By suppressing TNF-alpha and NF-kB, dimethyl sulfoxide (DMSO) blocks the production of damaging cytokines. The combination of shark cartilage, vitamin C, and DMSO has been reported to heal basal cell carcinoma.[308]

Glutamine

Studies suggest that glutamine—the most abundant amino acid in the human body—may decrease tumor progression.[309] It also may stabilize weight loss by allowing better nutrient absorption. The recommended dose is 2 g or more (not exceeding 14 g) daily.

ADDITIONAL SUPPLEMENTS

Dehydroepiandrosterone (DHEA)

Although dehydroepiandrosterone (DHEA) is naturally produced, we tend to produce less of this important hormone as we age. This decrease is connected to a number of degenerative conditions, including cancer.[310] Taking DHEA has been shown to reverse many illnesses including cancer, atherosclerosis, and diabetes.[311]

Melatonin

The pineal gland, located in the brain, produces this hormone, which not only is vital in regulating sleep cycles, as most of us have heard by now, but is immunity-enhancing as well. As with DHEA, levels of melatonin decrease as we age, so supplementation can be helpful. Melatonin increases the activity of our T-helper cells and aids our natural killer cells in getting rid of tumors. Supplements seem to extend the length of life, and the quality of life, in patients with inoperable brain tumors and metastatic gastric, colon, and breast cancer, as well as advanced endocrine tumors.[312, 313, 314, 315, 316] The suggested dose is 5 to 10 mg each night before bed.

Enzymes

Enzymes, which are catalysts for all life processes, are found in abundant supply in raw fruits and vegetables. Studies show that enzymes modulate inflammation, and that they may have a direct effect on controlling soft tissue cancers.[317, 318, 319, 320] Types of enzymes needed by cancer patients include trypsin, tyrotrypsin, pancreatin, bromelain (from pineapple), papain (from papaya), amylase, and lipase. The bioflavonoid rutin may be of additional benefit when combined with these enzymes.

Conjugated Linoleic Acid (CLA)

This trace fatty acid is extracted primarily from dairy products. It enhances apoptosis and blocks the growth and metastatic spread of tumors.[321, 322, 323] It suppresses arachidonic acid, which triggers inflammation. In combination with beta-carotene, CLA increases lymphocyte production and cytotoxicity. A relatively small dose (3–4 g) may prevent breast cancer. CLA has been observed to exert favorable effects on colorectal, lung, and prostate cancers in animal and in vitro studies.[324, 325, 326] For cancer patients, a dose of 1,000 mg of CLA six times per day is recommended. CLA should not be taken by women who are pregnant or lactating.

Modified Citrus Pectin

Modified citrus pectin (MCP) is a complex polysaccharide derived from the peel of citrus fruits. This substance is notable for its ability to bind to galectins—the membrane proteins on which cancer cells attach in order to metastasize—thereby inhibiting cancer cells from sticking together. MCP has been shown to impede the spread of prostate and other cancers.[327, 328, 329, 330] The typical adult dose of this soluble fiber is 6 to 30 g.

Lactoferrin

Lactoferrin is a milk protein that displays antibiotic, anti-inflammatory, and immunity-modulating properties by acting against the bacterium *Heliobacter pylori*, which induces gastritis, ulcers, and cancer. Lactoferrin has been observed to suppress angiogenesis and tumor metastasis in pancreatic, lung, and liver cancers.[331, 332, 333, 334] It also binds iron and scavenges free radicals in fluids and inflamed areas. Lactoferrin is found in the milk of cows, humans, sheep, and goats. It can be orally supplemented at a dosage of 300 to 900 mg per day.

N-Acetyl-Cysteine

N-acetyl cysteine, or NAC, reduces free radical damage in the body and helps metabolize carcinogens.[335, 336, 337, 338] This immunity-enhancer also helps prevent bladder hemorrhage from cancer drugs. The recommended dose is 2,000 mg per day.

Olive Leaf Extract

Known for its antimicrobial, antiviral, and antifungal properties, olive leaf extract is rich in antioxidants and is supportive of the immune system. The extract has been shown to help prevent skin cancer and induce cancer cell apoptosis.[339, 340, 341]

Shark Liver Oil

Shark liver oil contains alkyl glycerols, substances that have anti-tumor effects.[342, 343, 344] Studies show that when alkyl glycerols are given to women with uterine cancer prior to radium and X-ray therapy, the damage from these treatments is reduced.[345] A daily dose of 1,000 mg is suggested.

Resveratrol

This compound is one of the phytoalexins that are produced in plants during times of environmental stress, such as insect, animal, or pathogenic attack. Mulberries and the skins of red grapes are particularly rich in resveratrol. It is a very powerful antioxidant that provides greater protection against DNA damage than vitamins C or E or beta-carotene.

Resveratrol promotes healing by inhibiting the pro-inflammatory COX-2 enzyme. Studies demonstrate the ability of resveratrol to suppress tumor growth and block the formation of metastases.[346, 347, 348, 349, 350] The cellular development called differentiation is the process in which abnormal cells become more normal when cancerous cells start to destruct; resveratrol has the ability to promote such destruction. By inhibiting angiogenesis, resveratrol reduces tumor volume, weight, and metastasis. The suggested dose is 7 to 50 mg per day.

Bindweed

A growing body of research points to a common garden weed, bindweed, as a powerful inhibitor of tumor progression.[351] Studies show that the anticancer proteoglycan molecules (PGMs) in bindweed inhibit tumor growth in animals by 70 to 99.5 percent.[352]

Zinc

Zinc provides the body with a wide range of immune system functions. It supports the T and B cells in fighting infection and producing antibodies and works to promote healing and reduce infection. Studies have linked high dietary intake of zinc with a decreased risk of prostate cancer.[353, 354]

Chromium

This mineral acts like a hormone in the body in that it helps regulate our blood sugar levels. When blood sugar is normalized, immune function, and hence cancer resistance, is improved. This is why chromium supplements may be helpful in the prevention and treatment of cancer.

Genistein

Along with daidsein, genistein is a phytoestrogen from legumes that has antioxidant, anti-"bad" estrogen, and antitumor properties.[355, 356] The suggested dose for cancer patients is five 700 mg capsules four times per day of a soy extract that provides a minimum of 40 percent isoflavones. For prevention, 135 mg of 40 percent soy isoflavone extract once per day may be helpful.

HERBS

Herbs can help the immune system in three ways. They can stimulate immune defense reactions, suppress immune overreaction, and stimulate specific functions for short periods of time. The following herbs have multiple benefits, and are particularly noteworthy for their anticancer properties.

Aloe Vera

Aloe vera is antiseptic, antimicrobial, and anti-inflammatory. It supplies the system with amino acids and minerals, such as calcium, copper, iron, phosphorus, potassium, and zinc. Aloe vera contains live enzymes, including amylase, lactic dehydrogenase, and lipase, as well as the essential fatty acids needed for optimum health. Its role in treating tumors, research shows, is due to its ability to stimulate phagocytic activity.[357, 358, 359]

Astragalus

Although new to the West, astragalus is a time-honored Chinese remedy. In fact, traditional Chinese medical literature from 4,000 years ago says that astragalus has the ability to strengthen resistance to disease. Modern scientific research confirms these claims, demonstrating that not only does astragalus inhibit tumor growth but cells damaged by cancer and radiation are stimulated to full function with the introduction of this herb.[360, 361, 362, 363] Astragalus is considered a life energy, or qi tonic, that strengthens vitality and increases white blood cell and phagocytic activity. It is safe to take on a daily basis, making it an ideal preventative tonic. The recommended dose is 200 mg twice per day.

Ginkgo Biloba

This antioxidant herb, long used by the Chinese, works to counter a substance in the body called platelet activation factor, or PAF, which may act to encourage tumor growth. Laboratory studies demonstrate that gingko may be helpful in fighting ovarian, gastric, and other cancers.[364, 365, 366] Patients should take 125 mg three times daily.

Echinacea

When taken for short periods, echinacea revs up the immune system, stimulating the production and mobilization of white blood cells. It also stimulates cells in the lymphatic system, as well as important immune compounds, including interferon and tumor necrosis factor. Due to its immunosupportive properties, echinacea holds promise as a complementary alternative medicine for cancer patients.[367]

Garlic

There are numerous advantages to taking garlic, including anticancer benefits. Garlic makes cancer more recognizable to the immune system and interferes with the beginnings of tumor development. In addition, it stimulates immunity against formed tumor cells. Studies have observed a link between garlic and decreased risk of colon, lung, and stomach cancers.[368, 369, 370] Research suggests that the compound s-allyl cysteine, which is found in fresh garlic, helps decrease damage to organs resulting from chemotherapy.[371]

Ginger

Ginger will alleviate nausea associated with chemotherapy. It can be taken as a tea, or a small (0.5–1 inch) cube can be added to 10 ounces of juice. Scientific literature indicates that the anti-inflammatory properties of ginger are helpful in combating a variety of cancers.[372, 373, 374]

Turmeric

Part of the ginger family and an ingredient in curry powder, turmeric—or its main active component, curcumin—is a powerful antioxidant that produces a favorable effect on no fewer than ten causative factors in cancer development.[375] The compounds in this superfood have been shown to combat several types of cancer, including lung, breast, uterine, and colon cancer.[376, 377, 378, 379, 380, 381, 382] Curcumin inhibits COX-2 directly. It has also has anti-inflammatory effects, and it is known that chronic inflammation is the cause of colon cancer. Curcumin also inhibits, and even reverses, oxidative damage, and it protects DNA. To increase bioavailability, a small amount of piperine should be added. The normal dose is 900 mg daily, but cancer patients can take as many as four 900 mg capsules three times per day for a six- to twelve-month period. *Caution*: This herb should not be used in large quantities due to the potential for negative gastrointestinal side effects.

Ginseng

Studies associate the use of ginseng with lower incidences of numerous forms of cancer.[383, 384, 385] It contains ingredients called saponins that encourage macrophage and natural killer cell activity.

Theanine

This is a component of green tea that is structurally similar to glutathione, and its presence confuses cancer cells. Glutathione acts by blocking the ability of cancer cells to neutralize cancer-killing agents, resulting in the death of the tumor cell. Animal studies show that theanine has an antitumor effect and may improve the results of chemotherapy treatment.[386, 387, 388] The suggested dose is 500 to 1,000 mg daily, taken with doxorubicin.

Lentinan

This extract of the shiitake mushroom acts as an immune modulator and can help reduce the side effects of chemotherapy. Peer-reviewed journals report that lentinan also helps combat colorectal, stomach, and pancreatic cancers.[389, 390, 391, 392, 393]

Red Clover

Red clover checks free radical damage and protects DNA, which, in turn, helps prevent mutations.

Essiac

Taken in tea form, Essiac is an herbal formula that has been used for years to fight cancer. Among its immune-enhancing ingredients are burdock, Indian rhubarb, sheep sorrel, and slippery elm.

Hoxsey Herbal Therapy

Lymphoma and skin cancer have responded well to treatment with this herbal formula, which contains red clover, buckthorn bark, stillingia root, barberry bark, chaparral, licorice root, cascara amarga, and prickly ash bark, along with potassium iodide.

Berberine-Containing Herbs

These herbs include goldenseal, barberry, goldthread, and Oregon grape. Berberine inhibits an enzyme prominently involved in cancer formation. It is a potent antitumor agent because of its apoptosis-enhancing effect.[394, 395, 396] The suggested dose of goldenseal is 250 mg three times per day.

Feverfew

This is an anti-inflammatory herb that inhibits the production of several potentially damaging cytokines. Scientific literature has established feverfew's antiproliferative effects.[397, 398, 399] The suggested dose is one to two capsules per day that contain 600 mcg-parthenolide.

Other anticancer herbs to consider include African cayenne, bilberry, bloodroot, comfrey, dandelion root, goldenseal, paud'arco, and suma. Goldenseal should be taken for short periods of time, and not taken during pregnancy.

WHAT TO AVOID

Meat

Meat should be avoided, period. The saturated fat, excessive protein, bacteria, viruses, antibiotics, and hormones in meat are extremely harmful, and this is especially true of meat from animals raised on factory farms, because these animals are given high levels of antibiotics and hormones. Estrogenic compounds are routinely injected into commercially raised animals to fatten them up. Once eaten, these hormones are stored in estrogen-responsive tissue, whether it be ovarian, breast, testicular, or prostatic, where they overstimulate the body's own hormones and lead to cancer. If you must eat meat, consuming small quantities from animals raised naturally is a safer alternative.

Dairy Products

Dairy products contain ever-larger amounts of estrogen, thanks to bovine growth hormone and the fact that we now milk cows while they are pregnant. This excessive estrogen is harmful and promotes inflammation. One reason Japanese women do not get breast cancer as frequently as American women do may be that milk is not a staple of the Japanese diet. The consumption of dairy products promotes inflammation and taxes the immune system. High dietary intake has been linked with higher incidence of prostate, ovarian, breast, and other cancers.[400, 401, 402, 403]

Antibiotics

Antibiotics not only are overprescribed for us; they are regularly injected into livestock and thus become part of the food we eat. These drugs adversely affect the immune system by diminishing white blood cells needed to fight disease.[404]

Pesticides

In the 1960s, science writer Rachel Carson alerted the world to the damaging properties of pesticides in her highly acclaimed book *Silent Spring*. Sadly, the world has not heeded her warning and is paying dearly for it.

Numerous studies have linked indoor and outdoor pesticide use with increases in childhood leukemia and melanoma.[405, 406, 407] Common pesticide ingredients such as chlordane, heptachlor, Diazinon, and chlorpyrifos are associated with lymphomas, brain tumors, and non-Hodgkin's lymphoma.[408, 409] Pesticides can be avoided by steering clear of toxic household insecticides and consuming properly cleaned and peeled organic produce.

Tobacco

Everyone knows that smoking is a prime cause of the most prevalent form of cancer, lung cancer. More people are becoming aware of the dangers of secondhand smoke. Studies now confirm that 17 percent of lung cancers occur in people exposed to secondhand smoke between the ages of three and fifty but who have never smoked themselves. Cervical cancer is also associated with the inhalation of secondhand smoke. Chewing tobacco is not a good alternative to smoking, as it can lead to mouth cancer.

Alcohol

While drinking two to three alcoholic beverages weekly is considered moderate drinking in some circles, this amount has been associated with a significantly increased risk of breast cancer (one drink is considered to be 12 ounces of beer, 4 ounces of wine, or 1.5 ounces of hard liquor).[410, 411]

Radiation

X-rays should be taken only when absolutely necessary, as even low level exposure has been linked to cancer.[412] In addition, radiation from overexposure to sunlight can cause skin cancer.

Electromagnetic Radiation (EMR)

According to studies, people living close to high-tension wires are more likely to develop cancer than the general population.[413, 414, 415] Low level emissions of electromagnetic radiation from these wires over long periods of time are responsible. Electrical workers have an especially high rate of leukemia,[416] as do schoolchildren whose schools are near high-tension wires.[417] In the home, EMR comes from all appliances powered by electricity, such as televisions, computers, microwave ovens, electric blankets, and digital clocks. It is therefore important to unplug these items before going to sleep if they face the bed, even when they are behind a wall.

Processed Foods

Processed foods make up a large part of the standard American diet. These foods are lacking in critical micronutrients and fiber and only impair the body's ability to heal itself. Processed products are commonly made with damaging trans fat, and have high sugar and sodium contents. Replace processed foods with a diet of fresh and organic fruits, vegetables, grains, beans, legumes, and limited amounts of healthy fats, with an emphasis on raw foods. When cooking, never fry foods, as this produces a dangerous amount of potent carcinogens known as acrylamides.

Whole-Body
Approaches

Whole-body therapies involve a combination of approaches to cancer treatment and prevention, including diet and nutrition, herbs, immune enhancement, and detoxification. The following section highlights some whole-body therapies that I have found to be safe, effective, and natural.

Gerson Therapy

An ever-increasing number of toxic substances are introduced into the environment each year, ranging from chemicals, pesticides, and drugs to the byproducts of nuclear weapons and energy. Meanwhile, new agricultural and manufacturing techniques such as genetically engineered microorganisms and food irradiation alter the food we eat in ways that have not been evaluated. Until relatively recently, the human body, which has evolved over thousands of years, seemed to do a fairly good job of adapting to changes within the environment. Within the past century, however, the rate at which people have been exposed to new and toxic substances has accelerated so rapidly that the result has been a breakdown in the body's natural adaptation and defense processes. Certain physicians view this breakdown as one of the major contributing factors to many of today's most dreaded diseases, especially cancer. The theory that cancer is triggered by environmental factors that deplete the body's natural immunity and defense capabilities is not new. In fact, the late Dr. Max Gerson took an "environmental" approach to cancer therapy more than seventy years ago. The cornerstone of Dr. Gerson's therapy is detoxification of the body through diet designed to rehabilitate the body's natural immunity and healing processes.

Although Dr. Gerson died in 1959, his work has been carried on since that time by his daughter, Charlotte Gerson. Charlotte contracted bone tuberculosis (TB) at the age of eleven while fleeing Nazi Germany with her family, but was later cured by her father of this normally fatal disease. Vowing that Dr. Gerson's work would not die with him, Charlotte founded the Gerson Institute, which operates in two clinics: One is located along the western coast of Mexico about thirty minutes south of San Diego, and the other is near Budapest, Hungary. Dr. Gerson was eulogized by renowned physician and missionary Dr. Albert Schweitzer, whose wife Gerson cured of lung tuberculosis in the 1930s. Schweitzer wrote in a letter to Ms. Gerson,

> I see in him one of the most eminent geniuses in the history of medicine. Many of his basic ideas have been adopted without having his name connected with them. Yet he has achieved more than seemed possible under adverse conditions. He leaves a legacy which commands attention and which will assure him his due place. Those whom he cured will now attest to the truth of his ideas.[418]

The Discovery

Dr. Gerson was born in Germany in 1881. The roots of his work date to his early days as a young intern and resident before World War I. At that time he was suffering from severe migraine headaches, which were considered incurable. After a fruitless search through the medical literature, Dr. Gerson turned to nutrition to change his body chemistry and gain relief. He was already convinced that contamination of foods by artificial fertilizers and processing had a deleterious effect on the body and felt that he might be able to improve his migraine condition by restoring normal metabolism through a healthy diet. Gerson started to experiment on himself with certain foods in a meticulously detailed scientific study. His first experiment involved consuming nothing but cow's milk. Gerson reasoned that milk, being the first food, was something that even a baby could handle, so his body should have been able to utilize it properly. But when the milk diet made his headaches worse, it occurred to Dr. Gerson that milk is not normally consumed by adult animals other than humans anywhere in nature, and that perhaps milk is a foreign substance rather than a natural nutrient in the adult human diet.

Dr. Gerson decided to conduct his next experiments using foods that were more suited for the human type of build and body chemistry—namely, fruits and vegetables. (Contrary to popular belief, human physiology is basically herbivorous and not carnivorous. The human intestinal tract measures thirty feet in length and as such is unsuited to the proper digestion and elimination of meat, and our teeth are flat for grinding, not long, sharp, and pointed for ripping flesh.) Dr. Gerson found that he did not experience migraines when he ate nothing but grains, fresh fruits, and vegetables. He then began experimenting with single foods to discern their particular effect on his physiology. He found, for instance, that cooked foods often did not agree with him. It turned out to be the added salt, not the cooking process, that made the difference; when he ate the same cooked foods without salt, he was able to handle them very well.

Little by little, Dr. Gerson began to piece together a menu of foods that he could safely consume, as well as a list of foods that would regularly induce migraines within a few minutes of eating. He ultimately arrived at a diet very high in fresh fruits and vegetables and freshly prepared vegetable and fruit juices and very low in fats. Later, in his treatment of tuberculosis patients, Dr. Gerson would use a small amount of raw, fresh, unsalted butter because it is a good source of the phospholipids that form an important part of the body's defense mechanism. Otherwise the diet was largely free of animals fats, especially cooked fats, and totally free of meats and cooked animal proteins of any sort.

By the early 1920s, Dr. Gerson had succeeded in completely curing himself of migraines with his special diet. He then started extending his findings to patients who came to him suffering from migraines. They too benefited.

Eventually, although by accident, Dr. Gerson began to use his "Migraine Diet" in the treatment of tuberculosis as well. His daughter, Charlotte, relates how this occurred:

> One time, a patient came to him suffering from migraines and was given what he called his "Migraine Diet." When the patient came back after three or four weeks, he told Dr. Gerson that along with his migraines, he also had been suffering from lupus vulgaris, a form of skin tuberculosis, and that with the diet, not only had his migraines disappeared; the lupus had also begun to heal. Dr. Gerson found this almost impossible to believe, because he had learned that lupus was really an incurable condition. But there was the proof before his eyes. He saw that the lesion was healing, and he verified that it had been properly diagnosed and that there had been bacteriological studies showing that, in fact, the man had skin tuberculosis.[419]

Following this episode, Dr. Gerson was able to cure many other patients with skin tuberculosis. This therapy was later verified in large experiments in Munich, involving 450 terminal or incurable cases of skin tuberculosis treated with his Gerson dietary therapy. The treatment was shown to cure 447. From there, Dr. Gerson felt that if skin tuberculosis could be influenced by nutrition, why shouldn't other forms of tuberculosis respond? He applied this same dietary treatment to people with lung tuberculosis, bone tuberculosis, kidney tuberculosis, and other forms. One of the most famous patients he had at that time was the wife of Albert Schweitzer, who had contracted TB in the tropics. Her condition worsened when she was in a prisoner of war camp with her husband during the last part of World War I. The doctors had given up on Mrs. Schweitzer because her TB had spread to both lung fields and was quite extensive. But following Gerson's nutritional therapy, she recovered and lived another forty years, until passing away at age seventy-eight.

As a result of this healing, Drs. Gerson and Schweitzer became friends and remained so throughout their lives. Dr. Schweitzer followed the progress of the Gerson therapy as it was later applied to a wide variety of diseases. When he developed adult diabetes, Dr. Schweitzer found relief through Dr. Gerson's treatment. Unfortunately, the U.S. medical establishment has never shared Dr. Schweitzer's high opinion of Dr. Gerson. Instead of being praised, he was persecuted and harassed. Today, more than fifty years after Dr. Gerson's death in 1959, his therapy remains on the American Cancer Society's list of "Unproven Methods."

The Treatment

Before discussing Dr. Gerson's therapy, it is important to look at its theoretical basis. Like other alternative cancer approaches, Gerson therapy differs fundamentally from the traditional medical treatment, in that it deals with cancer as a systemic disease rather than a localized one. More specifically, Dr. Gerson's therapy aims to rebalance and revitalize the cancer patient's entire physiology in order to rectify this systemic disorder, thereby causing the cancer to regress and preventing it from recurring.

The core of Gerson therapy is a regimen consisting primarily of a salt- and fat-free diet of organically grown fresh fruits and vegetables that are usually served raw or as juices. The primary objective of the diet is to detoxify the body and rebalance the whole metabolism, rather than simply to eliminate the symptoms of the disease. "The treatment has to penetrate deeply to correct all vital processes," said Dr. Gerson. "When general metabolism is restored, we can again influence the functioning of all organs, tissues, and cells though it."[420]

Liver Therapy

Dr. Gerson placed particular importance on the condition of the liver, which is a primary regulator of metabolism. According to Dr. Gerson,

> The problem of the liver was and still is partly misunderstood and partly neglected. The metabolism and its concentration in the liver should be put in the foreground, not the cancer as a symptom. There, the outcome of cancer is determined as the clinically favorable results, failures, and autopsies clearly demonstrate. There the sentence will be passed—whether the tumors can be killed, dissolved, absorbed, or eliminated, and, finally, whether the body can be restored. The progress of the disease depends on whether and to what extent the liver can be restored.[421]

The liver's many functions, coupled with its constant interaction with the other organs of the body, give it a crucial role to play in the maintenance of health. Dr. Gerson and many other scientists have noted that in all degenerative diseases, including cancer, there are varying degrees of liver dysfunction and deterioration. Fortunately, however, the liver is not easily destroyed. While liver damage may not even be detected until liver function has been greatly impaired, the liver is also one of the organs that has the greatest capacity for regeneration. Consequently, restoration of the liver is a significant objective of Dr. Gerson's diet.

Dr. Gerson's liver therapy is multifaceted. First, animal proteins are eliminated or greatly reduced in the diet because they have been found to interfere with liver therapy and impede the body's detoxification. The ideal diet for patients on liver therapy, as mentioned above, is low in salt and fat, and high in potassium and fresh fruits and vegetables, mostly in juice form. The juice is always prepared freshly and is not mixed with other medications that could alter the pH and thereby decrease its efficacy. Restoration of the liver, which may take from six to eighteen months, depending on the severity of the illness, allows the liver to detoxify the body and produce its own oxidative enzymes.

Other aspects of liver therapy include liver injections, and lubile (defatted bile powder from young calves) and pancreatin (pancreatic enzyme) tablets. The liver injections are composed of liver extract and are given daily for four to six months. They, too, provide important vitamins, minerals, and enzymes that aid in restoring the liver to its proper functioning. These liver injections are usually combined with vitamin B12 injections, which Dr. Gerson believed are important for proper protein synthesis. Cancer patients are often unable to combine amino acids properly in order to form proteins within their bodies. Lubile was used more frequently in the earlier stages of the therapy. While it is not used for most patients today, it is beneficial in cases where the liver is extremely damaged and the bile duct system is impaired. Pancreatin tablets are given during and after the detoxification program as a backup source of digestive enzymes, because those are also deficient in most cancer patients.

According to Dr. Gerson, patients on the therapy actually begin to break down, assimilate, and eliminate cancer tumors. This is accomplished when the repaired liver is adequately producing oxidative enzymes, the general detoxification process (of which the liver is a critical part) is active, and potassium levels throughout the body are adequate.

Coffee Enemas

During the period when the body is killing, absorbing, and eliminating the tumor, detoxification is of the utmost importance. Dr. Gerson admitted that in the early stages of development, the therapy did not contain adequate detoxification techniques. "After a tumor was killed," he says, "the patient did not die of cancer but of a serious intoxication with 'coma hepaticum' (liver shock) caused by absorption of necrotic cancer tissue."[422] Thus, in addition to the other cleansing aspects of the therapy, Dr. Gerson began to prescribe frequent coffee enemas, which at the outset of treatment can be given as often as every four hours. This prescription derives from the work of two German researchers who found that caffeine administered rectally causes the bile ducts to open, instigating an increased production of bile, which flushes out the accumulated toxins.

After these enemas, Dr. Gerson noticed that patients were often relieved of pain (e.g., headaches), fevers, and nausea, which allowed him to then easily discontinue their pain medication and sedation. On the other hand, Dr. Gerson noted that coffee taken orally seemed to have exactly the opposite effect: It caused the stomach to go into spasm and produce a "soaping" over or contraction of the bile ducts. Hence, while regular coffee enemas are an indispensable part of Gerson therapy, drinking coffee is discouraged.

Reestablishing Potassium Levels

Muscles, the brain, and the liver normally have much higher levels of potassium than sodium. Early in his research, however, Dr. Gerson noted that this ratio is reversed in cancer patients; that is, he found that sodium is elevated in cancer cells and that in the ailing body, potassium is often inactive and/or improperly utilized. He felt that chronic disease is initiated by the loss of potassium from the cell system. Accordingly, another primary objective of Gerson therapy is to reestablish proper levels of potassium in the body. Because of the specific relationship between sodium and potassium, in which an increase in one mineral causes a decrease in the other and vice versa, one of the first actions Dr. Gerson advocated was the elimination of salt and sodium-rich foods from the diet. In addition, all patients on Gerson therapy immediately begin receiving large amounts of a potassium solution that Dr. Gerson developed after 300 experiments. The potassium compound he used, which is still used at the Gerson clinics, is a combination of potassium gluconate, potassium acetate, and potassium phosphate monobasic. This is administered in the form of a 10 percent potassium solution, which is added to juices ten times daily in 4-teaspoon doses. The potassium solution is never added to the liver juice, because Dr. Gerson believed that it can alter the juice's pH, thereby decreasing its efficacy. After a month, the amount is decreased by about half. The fluid retention and edema (caused by a sodium overabundance) is usually the first thing to disappear when patients are given high amounts of potassium in juices. Dr. Gerson noted that even in a healthy person it is very difficult to restore potassium deficiencies. It may take as long as a year or two before normal levels in major organs are reestablished in seriously ill people. In patients suffering from dehydration, potassium is added to the fluids therapeutically administered in the form of a GKI (glucose, potassium, insulin) solution. According to Charlotte Gerson, this solution is not specific to Gerson therapy but is recognized and utilized by the American medical establishment in general. "Dr. Demetrio Sodi-Pallares, a world-renowned cardiologist from Mexico City," says Ms. Gerson, "very much recommends this solution."[423] He agrees with Dr. Gerson that disease is systemic or metabolic. His own research in heart disease has shown that it is not a disease of the heart but a metabolic disease that must be treated with a high-potassium, low-sodium diet.[424] Dr. Sodi-Pallares found that giving GKI to heart patients with fluid retention is also very helpful. Ms. Gerson noted, "This solution helps restore potassium to the cell system. Energy is required in order for potassium to go back into the cell system, and this energy is supplied by the glucose and insulin. We use this solution quite successfully in two ways: first to replenish the patient with fluids, but also to restore potassium to the cells and reduce edema."

Diet

Every aspect of Gerson therapy revolves around the diet, which is designed to support all the other efforts to rebalance the internal body chemistry. At the clinics, all meals are prepared with fresh, organically grown produce. Nothing is canned, jarred, pickled, frozen, or preserved in any way. Between the juices and the meals, the total average intake of food for each patient is approximately 20 pounds of fresh raw food per day, mostly via juices. All refined, processed, and empty-calorie foods are avoided. This includes obviously treated foods such as white sugars and flours, and smoked, sulfured, packaged, or mass-prepared products. Other obvious taboos include cigarettes, alcohol, drugs, and caffeine, which are known to deplete the immune system and act as carcinogens. All animal proteins such as meat, poultry, and dairy products are avoided, because they are difficult to digest and hinder, rather than promote, the restoration of the liver.

Both animal and vegetable fats are also avoided, as they too can be difficult to digest and can impede detoxification. In addition, Dr. Gerson found that dietary fats actually have the effect of promoting tumor growth. This accords with cancer research indicating that the higher the level of cholesterol and fats in the blood of cancer patients, the less their chance of surviving. Dr. Gerson slowly eliminated all fats from the diets of his cancer patients and found that the results improved substantially. On the other hand, whenever he added fats (even oils that are low in cholesterol) to the patients' diets, he observed regrowth of tumor tissue. Consequently, for cancer patients receiving Gerson therapy, fats of animal and vegetable origin are eliminated as much as possible. The only exception is linseed oil, which Dr. Gerson found is particularly well tolerated. (For patients suffering from other illnesses, while the diet is still essentially low in fat, some raw fresh butter, egg yolks, and low-cholesterol vegetable oils such as safflower oil and sunflower oil may be eaten in small quantities.)

Dr. Gerson was a strong believer in the importance of organically grown produce, and, as mentioned previously, all food used at his clinic must be grown in this manner. Chemical pesticides and fertilizers, he said, essentially poison and denature fruits and vegetables by altering their chemical composition. For instance, he found that many chemical fertilizers cause the sodium content in the affected foods to rise while decreasing potassium levels, which is precisely contrary to what the body requires to restore healthy metabolic function.

The "Healing Crisis"

A "healing crisis" is an activation of the body's defenses, and often takes the form of fever as the immune system begins to be functional again. Ms. Gerson says,

> Almost invariably, once the patient begins to produce a fever, this is followed by a tumor reduction. It seems as though the fever helps the body break down and dissolve the tumor tissue. Along with the fever come flulike symptoms such as aches and pains all over the body. This healing crisis can be quite severe in cases where the body is getting rid of accumulated heavy toxic materials. These toxins are removed through the coffee enemas, but sometimes the patient will have a very irritated colon because these materials literally burn as they are being released. In those cases, we alter from the coffee to chamomile tea enemas, which are soothing and help the body release toxic materials which have built up. We see that type of problem with patients who have been medicated a lot with tranquilizers and antidepressants. The latter are especially toxic. When they have been used a fair amount, the patients suffer a lot as they are released from the body. We have to give these patients chamomile tea enemas, peppermint tea and chamomile tea by mouth, and oatmeal gruel—all are soothing.

Usually these reactions last no longer than three to four days, and when they are over, the patients claim to be much relieved and improved, with a better appetite. Sometimes, if patients have experienced a good deal of weight loss, they become ravenously hungry. This is part of the body's normal healing process. Ms. Gerson tells of a thirty-eight-year-old patient with liver and pancreatic cancer who had been told on October 1 that she would not survive past Christmas. She was on twelve morphine tablets per day and had lost twenty-five pounds. In two days she was free of pain and off the morphine, then went through a healing crisis with fever, came out of it after about six or seven days, and started to be very hungry. Every time she went to dinner, she took food back to her room so that she could have an extra meal or two in the middle of the night. This patient not only survived past Christmas but told Ms. Gerson years later that she was feeling wonderful and had resumed most of her normal activities.

The Patients

Cancer patients have been treated with Gerson therapy for more than sixty years, and the results have been amazing, especially in contrast to those reported by conventional cancer specialists and agencies. The therapy was administered at treatment centers in New York and then California before the establishment of the new Gerson Therapy Center in Mexico in 1977. Currently, the California-based Gerson Institute licenses two private clinics: the Clinica Nutrición y Vida in Tijuana, Mexico, and the Gerson Health Centre near Budapest, Hungary, which opened in 2009. The Clinica Nutrición y Vida accommodates around 130 patients each year, while the Budapest clinic cares for approximately sixty patients. At any given time, thousands of cancer patients self-administer Gerson therapy at home, but the Gerson Institute is unable to estimate how many home patients there are. A treatment at the Tijuana clinic usually lasts around three weeks and costs $5,500 per patient. The cost includes room and board for one companion to the patient.

A 40 to 50 percent improvement rate was recorded in terminal patients, and an 80 percent improvement in early to moderate cancer cases.[425] A study reviewing the effectiveness of treating melanoma patients with Gerson therapy compared to conventional treatments concluded that reports of five-year survival were "considerably higher than those reported elsewhere," and that "stage III A/B males had exceptionally high survival rates compared with those reported by other centers."[426] For more information on this therapy, contact:

> Gerson Institute
> (800) 838-2256
> www.gerson.org

THE ISSELS TREATMENT (FORMERLY KNOWN AS *GANZHEIT* THERAPY)

Trained as a traditional surgeon, the late German physician Dr. Joseph Issels was widely regarded as the father of integrative medicine, combining alternative and complementary medicine decades before its current popularity. Issels became aware of the limitations of orthodox therapy when he began treating cancer patients and found that the survival rate was frustratingly low. His observations convinced him that the successful treatment of cancer required a return to the whole-body (or *Ganzheit*) approach to the disease. Issels strongly believed that "cancer is not just a local disease confined to the particular place in the body where the tumor manifests itself but is a general disease of the whole body."[427] Convinced of the body's inherent ability to heal itself, Dr. Issels developed a broad-spectrum therapy to restore and regenerate the body's natural defense mechanisms, which complements traditional Western medical treatment directed at the elimination of a localized tumor. With this approach, Dr. Issels achieved a degree of success in treating his cancer patients that is unparalleled in traditional medicine, ultimately demonstrating the most successful results ever achieved with late-stage cancer patients—16.6 percent five-year survival and 15 percent fifteen-year survival.

The Discovery

How did it all begin? In his early years of medicine, Dr. Issels put some of his theories into practice in what he would later call a *"Ganzheit"* or "whole-body" approach to healing. He required that his patients have infected teeth or tonsils removed, because he strongly believed that chronic bacterial infection can release poisons into the body that lower natural resistance and trigger disease. Proper diet was also considered critical. The usual foodstuffs had to be replaced with biologically adequate ones adjusted to fit the organic conditions of individual patients, but all diets were based on whole, organic plant foods. Chronically ill patients usually had to receive lactobacillus acidophilus, a cultured milk product that served as a ferment substitute to compensate for a loss of efficiency in their digestive systems. Tobacco, alcohol, coffee, tea, and other substances the doctor considered harmful were banned. Whenever possible, longstanding emotional stress was relieved or eliminated. In the meantime, the doctor went ahead with treatment of the particular diseased organ, confident that he was also addressing the root cause of the patient's sickness.

Initially, Issels's success at curing cancer or achieving long-term remission was not great. He knew that his colleagues were equally baffled by the disease, but that knowledge did not ease his frustration. Surgery and radiation seemed to bring temporary improvement, but it was clear that they did not get at the cause of the cancer and could not protect the patient from further occurrences. Surely, Dr. Issels thought, there had to be a way of applying the principles of *Ganzheit* therapy to the treatment of cancer to produce not just remissions but genuine cures. There had to be an alternative to disfiguring surgery, toxic chemicals, and poisonous radiation.

Dr. Issels was soon getting remarkable results with this combination of *Ganzheit* therapy, homeopathy, dietary control, and other therapeutic techniques. His practice became the largest in town, but because of his compassion for cancer sufferers and a willingness to provide treatment for low or no cost, the practice did not make him a rich man.

Using History as a Guide

The antipathy Dr. Issels had felt toward cancer in his early years became almost an obsession with the disease. He read everything he could find on cancer and in the process became an expert in medical history. He discovered to his surprise that cancer, contrary to popular opinion, was not a modern affliction but had been observed by Chinese and Sumerian physicians and described in manuscripts dating back 3,000 years BCE. Even that long ago, cancer was thought to result from a malfunction in the body's regulatory mechanisms and was treated with acupuncture and drugs.

Hippocrates (460–377 BCE), the founder of Western medicine, was the first to use the word "carcinoma" in referring to malignant tumors, which he believed arose from a "separation of the humors" (blood, bile, and phlegm) and was to be treated with surgery and drugs. But what Dr. Issels found especially noteworthy was Hippocrates' recommendation that the entire body be detoxified and that cancer patients be put on a special diet, much like his own *Ganzheit* theory. Further research showed that for the ancient Greeks, *diata,* or "diet," referred to far more than what a patient was to eat or drink. The term was closer in meaning to "way of life" or "lifestyle" and strongly suggested abstinence from anything that might be spiritually as well as physically harmful.

The Roman physician Claudius Galen (131–200CE), the founder of scientific physiology, whose authority had gone unchallenged in Western medicine for over 1,000 years, had also turned his attention to cancer, as Dr. Issels soon discovered. Galen also held the opinion that cancer is a disease of the entire body, not confined to the site of the tumor.

Moving forward in time, Dr. Issels encountered the world-famous doctor of the Renaissance, Philippus Aureolus Theophrastus Bombastus von Hohenheim, better known as Paracelsus, who also felt that the physician's role in treating cancer and other diseases was not to interfere with the body but rather to stimulate the healing processes nature had provided to correct the imbalances in the body that result in illness. Dr. Issels also encountered the pioneer surgeon Ambroise Paré, who shared Paracelsus's view of cancer as a disease of the entire body, and the French thinker René Descartes, who thought cancer was caused by abnormalities in the lymph glands. He pored over the work of Percival Potts, the 18th-century British physician who was among the first to describe cancer as an "occupational" malignancy when he noticed an abnormally high rate of cancer of the scrotum in young chimney sweeps. In short, no one who might have something useful to say about cancer escaped Issels's scrutiny.

The work of Dr. Edward Jenner, the English physician who had developed a vaccination and checked the scourge of smallpox, seemed to offer special promise in regard to both theory and practice. Although Dr. Jenner had not been successful in treating cancer, he had produced vaccines that had shown promising results against other disorders. Equally important for Dr. Issels, his British predecessor believed that cancer stemmed from inadequacies in the immune mechanisms and that it could have a fatal effect only when the body's natural immunity had broken down completely.

Searching for a Vaccine

Following this line of thought, Dr. Issels searched for a vaccine that would bolster the body's immune system to the point where it could fight back successfully against cancer. Neoblastine, a vaccine he developed by culturing cancer tissues in a controlled medium many times over a long period to insure safety, seemed to offer some promise. After testing the vaccine on laboratory animals, he tried it on a terminally ill lung cancer patient, together with his *Ganzheit* therapy involving extraction of infected teeth and tonsils, and strict dietary control.

Although the patient lived three months longer than expected, the results were ambiguous, because there had been no cure and it was impossible to attribute the patient's improvement to any single factor in the treatment.

Another case, on the surface equally disappointing, occurred when Dr. Issels agreed to treat a woman with an enormous uterine tumor who had already been given up on by her doctors. Heeding her husband's pleas, Dr. Issels agreed to see her, but he could do nothing beyond prescribing painkillers and ordering a change in her diet. Nonetheless, the fact that Dr. Issels had undertaken to treat her gave the woman a much better outlook. Until her death two months later, she maintained steadfastly that Dr. Issels's treatments had freed her of pain that drugs had been unable to eliminate.

Issels became convinced that a tumor was merely a late-stage symptom, accidentally triggered but able to grow only in what he described as a "tumor milieu," the result of prior damage to organs and organ systems, especially those involved in maintaining the body's resistance to disease. The disease would never gain a foothold unless the body's defenses were depleted. Issels posited that once cancer had gained a foothold, conventional treatments could usually provide only temporary relief. While surgery, by removing large masses of tumor, might stimulate the immune system to regenerate, it was not likely to provide a cure by itself because the operation could not get at the underlying cause of the cancer. Radiation and chemotherapy, while initially successful, frequently provided only temporary relief. Nonetheless, Dr. Issels did not offer *Ganzheit* therapy as a substitute for the usual treatments, but as a supplement that he believed would make the conventional therapies more effective by rehabilitating the entire patient instead of just attacking the tumor.

Combining Traditional and Unconventional Methods

As the number of his cancer patients continued to grow, Dr. Issels began specializing in that disease. In 1950, he took charge of a thirty-bed cancer unit at a clinic in a small town in Bavaria. There, he put in seventeen-hour days, treating patients with a combination of traditional and unconventional methods. Surgery was used to remove large tumors. Drugs were administered to improve the functioning of various organs, especially the liver and kidneys, which usually are severely damaged in advanced cancer patients. The body was detoxified through the use of purifying drugs; mild purgatives; a diet high in fruit, vegetables, and grains; and the consumption of large amounts of water, juice, and herbal teas. Homeopathic remedies were used along with vaccines to stimulate antibody production.

Dr. Issels' treatment did not cure all cancer patients, but considering most of his patients were late- or end-stage in their disease, it was remarkable that he was able to extend life by months or years. Those who came to him were patients whom the medical establishment had been unable to help and had given up on. For them, Dr. Issels offered the proverbial "last, best, hope" of staying alive, a hope he was sometimes able to fulfill in ways that bordered on the miraculous.

The Treatment

Although about 90 percent of the patients he saw had already been designated as incurable and beyond the help of orthodox medicine,

Dr. Issels continued conventional treatment if it was possible and appropriate. He viewed *Ganzheit* therapy as a supplement to make these treatments more effective rather than as a substitute for them.

Tonsillectomy and Tooth Extraction

Under *Ganzheit* therapy, patients part with infected teeth and tonsils. Dr. Issels viewed these as sites of infection that place an unnecessary burden on the immune system and act to lower the body's general defenses against disease. Dental amalgams also are removed.

Diet and Nutrition

Diet is a critical component of *Ganzheit* therapy. Most meats are avoided, because meat is difficult for advanced cancer patients to digest and is usually filled with hormones, antibiotics, and pesticides that place further strain on the body. The recommended diet is primarily vegetarian, focusing on organically grown whole grains, fruits, and vegetables, supplemented by enzymes, minerals, and vitamins, with emphasis on A, B-complex, C, and E. Yogurt and acidophilus supplements are used to eliminate abnormal intestinal flora. Serum activator is administered to bring the metabolism of red blood cells up to normal levels, allowing the release of additional hemoglobin and thus increasing the supply of oxygen to the body's cells. Organ extracts are supplied to help repair secondary damage to organs and improve their functioning, while a high fluid intake backed up with herbal extracts is used to detoxify the body; improve kidney, lymph, and liver functions; and bolster the excretory systems.

Psychotherapy

Because *Ganzheit* therapy entails the treatment of the entire patient, individual and group psychotherapy is an important element. Through this treatment, Dr. Issels hoped not only to help the patient come to terms with the disease but also to alleviate or remove the psychic stress that he felt could help bring on cancer and hinder its cure.

Immunotherapy

A major component of the treatment is a highly sophisticated form of immunotherapy, geared specifically to fighting cancer and supported, where necessary, by surgery, radiation, and chemotherapy. This immunotherapy involves a twofold approach: specific immunization against the particular type of cancer and a general effort to augment the body's natural immune responses.

"Specific immunization works on a well-tried principle," Dr. Issels wrote in his 1975 book, *Cancer: A Second Opinion*. "Once a particular cancer antigen has been identified, it is administered under conditions most favorable for the induction of an immune response that will destroy cancer cells bearing that antigen. This is really no more than an extension of the standard vaccination technique against any infectious disease."

For specific immunization against the tumor, Dr. Issels often administered a vaccine developed by Viennese scientist Dr. Franz Gerlach, that was shown to cause regression of malignant tumors. Other tumor-specific immunization was effected with standard nontoxic vaccines such as Centanit for carcinoma, Sarkogen for sarcoma, and Lymphogran for Hodgkin's disease.

General immunotherapy is used to bolster the patient's overall immunity and to destroy the "tumor milieu" that makes it possible for the cancer to sustain itself and grow. Here the primary means of attack consists of autovaccines prepared from extracts from the patient's own teeth and tonsils as well as other nontoxic vaccines designed to boost general resistance to disease.

Ozone Therapy

Ozone therapy, although not a direct aid to the immune system, is also used as a means of increasing the oxygen supply to the cells and destroying viruses and bacteria in the bloodstream. This method of systematically exposing portions of the patient's blood supply to medically pure ozone is not commonly practiced in the United States, but has been used against blood-borne infectious diseases in Germany for more than twenty-five years. Dr. Issels found the therapy to be effective in purging the blood of oxidation-resistant pesticides and other toxins.

Hyperpyrexia (Fever Induction)

Hyperpyrexia, homeopathy's long-sanctioned induction of fever, is also used in much the same way as ozone therapy to make life uncomfortable for the tumor. Once a month patients get a "fever shot," which can raise the body temperature as high as 105 degrees Fahrenheit, where it stays for several minutes while the patient is under constant medical supervision.

While Dr. Issels may not have shared the enthusiasm of the ancient Greek physician who remarked, "Give me a chance to produce fever, and I can cure all illness," he knew that fever was a natural reaction of the body to foreign invaders and that it made these invaders more vulnerable to attack. He also discovered that the number of disease-destroying leukocytes (white blood cells) in the patient's bloodstream rose enormously after each fever shot and that the patients uniformly reported feeling much better afterward as their bodies were detoxified. Even localized heating of the tumor area, Dr. Issels discovered, could have effects which, while not as spectacular, were clearly beneficial.

The Results

Three independent studies of Dr. Issels' medical records conducted by highly reputed experts confirmed a 16.6 percent cure rate among the terminal patients treated with *Ganzheit* therapy. To understand the significance of this figure, it is necessary to recall that all these patients were terminal, already given up on by conventional medicine. In the United States, for example, such a patient has virtually no chance of survival, let alone of cure.

This distinction between survival and cure is also crucial. For conventional medicine, "cure" simply means that the cancer patient has survived five years after the initial diagnosis. It says nothing about the state of the patient during that time or at its end. Dr. Issels used a different standard.

While even Dr. Issels did not think of *Ganzheit* therapy as the perfect cure for cancer, his indisputable successes bring one face-to-face with some uncomfortable facts about the state of cancer treatment today. The tremendous technological advances in surgery, radiation, and chemotherapy have been of benefit to some cancer patients, but these benefits appear to have peaked in the mid-1950s. Notwithstanding the stunning array of new high-tech surgical procedures and chemotherapeutic drugs, traditional medicine has not been able to obtain more than a slight increase in the survival rates of patients, if that. Despite the expenditure of billions of dollars in the war on cancer, there is growing evidence of the limitations of conventional therapies and evidence that statistical manipulations have grossly inflated the amount of actual progress.

Dr. Issels continued his fight against cancer throughout his life. In the years before he died in 1998 at the age of ninety, Dr. Issels and colleagues at the Centro Hospitalario Internacional Pacifico, S.A. (CHIPSA) Center for Integrative Medicine refined a program that combined his comprehensive immunotherapy with the similarly holistic approach developed by the late Dr. Max Gerson, another leader in the alternative medicine field.

Issels Treatment is currently practiced at a clinic located in Santa Barbara, California, and another in Tijuana, Mexico. The average cost of the standard three-week treatment is $15,000 but can vary depending on the clinic location. For more information on this therapy, contact:

> The Issels Foundation
> (888) 447-7357
> www.issels.com

THE ECLECTIC TRIPHASIC MEDICAL SYSTEM (ETMS)

The Eclectic Triphasic Medical System (ETMS) was pioneered by Dr. Donald Yance, a practicing clinical herbalist, certified nutritionist, author of *Dietary, Herbal and Nutritional Strategies for Treating and Preventing Cancer*, and the founder of the Mederi Centre for Natural Healing. The ETMS approach to cancer incorporates both traditional and modern healing techniques, with an emphasis on herbal medicine. In an interview between Dr. Yance and myself, he describes his protocol for treating and preventing cancer:

> The foods that I would emphasize in general are first of all the highest quality attainable, as fresh as possible, and organic. I always stress quality and balance. I don't care if you think you should be juicing carrots, beets, and celery; in my opinion they must be organic and they must be fresh. I tend to base a lot of my specifics on the person's health status, the person's genetic makeup, and the type of cancer they have. Of course I am going to emphasize foods that contain a high level of phytochemicals that we know inhibit cancer and possibly can reverse cancer.
>
> Phytochemicals and phytonutrients are new terms that describe plant constituents that are not vitamins or minerals but various compounds that play an important role in cell protection. They protect against the initiation and promotion of cancer. Of the flavones, my favorite is called quercetin, which is found abundantly in broccoli and in onions and is a wonderful inhibitor of a number of different cancer cell lines. Isoflavones are found in the soybean food family. Tryterpines, limolines, and nomlines are found in citrus fruit, mostly in the rind and the oil of the citrus, which can be made into a tea with orange peel, lemon peel, or from the oils. Some of these are in clinical trials for cancer therapy.

Dr. Yance continues,

I am a big believer in Omega-3 fatty acids. Not only do they have strong inhibitory effects on cancer growth from many mechanisms, but they also help to feed the body nutrition-wise, particularly combined with protein. I know there are a lot of different viewpoints on this topic. Do I need to build up this person while at the same time detoxifying them? That is where you play the balance between foods that will build a person and inhibit cancer, and foods that will detoxify the person.

So a combination of detoxification and health-restoring diet is essential to Dr. Yance's approach.

Detoxification

Dr. Yance describes his detoxifying program:

I use Epsom salt baths, which do a number of things. First, you raise the thermal level of the core body temperature. Most people with cancer have a very subnormal body temperature. It is important to get the body's immune system activated by raising the body temperature. When people are in contact with some sort of pathogen, the body's natural response is to secrete pyrogens that raise the body's temperature. We do this artificially because cancer does not provoke the usual immunological reaction, so we do things to help that. I mix essential oils, mostly lavender, into the bathtub and give them an herbal compound along with an herbal tea. I also put a big emphasis on liver detoxifying, in which I will use a number of different plant compounds along with various supplements. I favor alpha-lipoic acid combined with some very concentrated forms of herbs, particularly turmeric. Alpha-lipoic acid is a highly absorbable nutrient that is both fat- and water-soluble. In my opinion it is the first precursor of glutathione, which is part of the phase II liver enzyme detoxifying system. It helps detoxify xenoestrogens, lipid soluble toxins, some other drugs and pollutants, and possibly some other things like dead cancer cells. The liver is the main vehicle for breaking these things down and helping the body secrete them. The dosage I use is 300 mg of lipoic acid twice per day.

As far as turmeric goes, I use a compound of standardized curcuminoids, the active constituent in turmeric, about 95 to 97 percent. I use 1 gram three or four times per day on an empty stomach combined with bromelain. Bromelain is an enzyme from pineapple that interacts with the turmeric and with quercetin. The dosages of quercetin and bromelain are the same, 1 gram three or four times per day on an empty stomach. These three compounds have a synergistic effect in that they all help each other be absorbed more efficiently.

Other Herbs

Dr. Yance tells us about some other commonly used herbs:

An interesting plant that I use quite a bit in breast cancer is an herb called pulsatilla, which has no anticancer activity but tends to lift a person's spirit. I think that ability is the first and foremost part of any person's treatment. Then we move on to plants like schisandra, known as a five-spice herb in Chinese medicine because it has salt, sweet, bitter, pungent, and sour taste all in one plant. It is a wonderful hepatic protective agent and detoxifier and also is used to treat nervous exhaustion. It helps the body's endocrine system with the stress of having cancer. It balances the pH of the digestive system, which may be too alkaline or too acidic, and so improves the ability of the body to absorb. It is perhaps the most powerful liver protective agent of all plants. Red clover is a wonderful plant particularly with some of the hormonal type cancers, like breast cancer and prostate cancer. Because of the isoflavones and curcuminoids present in this plant, I use a one-to-one extract of red clover instead of the over-the-counter preparations of one-to-five, which are not as strong. I make a decoction (a tea you prepare by boiling until the water is two-thirds evaporated and then straining before consumption) of blossoms of red clover, which is also very nice.

Licorice is also a wonderful plant. It has hormone-regulating properties and liver-protective properties; it is a demulcent, so it soothes mucus membranes; and it is a precursor to aldosterone. Aldosterone is the hormone that tells the body to hold onto fluids. If a person has very dry skin, and every time they drink liquid, they urinate it right out of their bodies, their blood pressure tends to be very low; they may have low levels of aldosterone, so think of using a little licorice.

Emotional and Spiritual Health

Attitude, love, and spirituality play a part in healing cancer, as in many other diseases. As Dr. Yance says,

I believe this is the essence of healing. It is difficult to give any kind of nutritional support until a person has their fear of the cancer removed. When they have fear, they have very poor quality of sleep. Sleep is essential for detoxification. The body does most of its detoxifying while it is in the deepest rest. Fear is an obstacle in the way of healing, and I believe this is where you tap into a person's spirit. Once a person is comfortable with who they are spiritually, they no longer have fear. The whole body, mind, and spirit are interrelated. When you feel comfortable with who you are spiritually you don't worry about things as much.

I always explain that we are all going to ultimately die. We need to come to grips with that and not fixate on it. Let's think about the living, let's think about today, let's think about how we can step forward and be healed, because you don't want to live miserably anyway. Let's think about how you can enrich yourself on all levels and that everything complements each other. One of my great loves for plant medicine is that plants are here on earth just like we are, and they exude a tremendous amount of healing. We have only scraped the iceberg of the ability of plants to heal.

Treatment Details

The typical cost of ETMS cancer treatment administered by Dr. Yance and his colleagues at the Mederi Centre for Natural Healing in Ashland, Oregon is $1,000 per month.

For more information on this therapy, contact

Mederi Centre for Natural Healing
(541) 488-3133
www.mederifoundation.org

ANTINEOPLASTON THERAPY

Forty years ago, a medical student in Poland took a new and different approach to cancer research. He decided to find out why all people don't have cancer. Everyone is exposed to the same known and unknown causative agents of this disease. What is different about the people who never contract it? Is this difference the key to developing a cure?

The Discovery: Dr. Stanislaw Burzynski

Dr. Stanislaw Burzynski believes so. Now working out of a research facility he founded in 1970 in Houston, Texas, Dr. Burzynski has successfully treated about 2,000 patients with advanced cancer.

119

Most of these people turned to him as a last resort when conventional treatment with radiation, chemotherapy, and surgery had failed. What they found was a therapy based not on the abuse of the body's built-in defense systems but rather on the transformation of cancerous cells into healthy, normal tissue.

Dr. Burzynski's solution lies in a group of chemical substances, part of a larger group of chemical compounds called peptides, which exist in every human body. His research points to a severe shortage of these substances—called antineoplastons—in cancer patients. Simply stated, antineoplastons are a special class of peptides, found in the body, that combat neoplastons—abnormal cells or cancer cells. Antineoplastons could be the vehicle needed by the body to ward off and even reverse the development of these cancerous cells. Dr. Burzynski has put this theory into action, treating patients by reintroducing antineoplastons into the bloodstream, either intravenously or orally with capsules. In many cases, tumors shrank in size or actually disappeared. Some patients even experienced complete remission of their cancers, and years of follow-up study have revealed no sign of any return.

Such results are almost unbelievable. Dr. Burzynski appears to have tapped the power of antineoplastons to naturally "reprogram" cancer cells. His approach could virtually eliminate the need to destroy these cells or remove the tumors they create. This therapy was not developed overnight. It took Dr. Burzynski nearly three decades of research, first in Poland, then at the Baylor College of Medicine in Houston, Texas, and ultimately at the Burzynski Research Institute in Houston. During this time, Dr. Burzynski zeroed in on the substance he named "antineoplaston." But to get back to Dr. Burzynski's original concern, why do tumors develop in the first place?

Why Tumors Develop

According to Burzynski's theory, cancer is caused primarily by an information-processing error. Good information produces healthy cells; bad information results in cancerous cells. Antineoplastons are important because they carry "good" information to the cells. They can "tell" the cells to develop normally.

All cells start out with specific goals. Some turn into skin, some into blood vessels, some into bone or other body tissues. However, they will never go on to perform these highly specialized functions in the body unless they go through a process called *differentiation*. Cancer cells, or neoplastons, which everybody produces regularly, never differentiate. They are abnormal cells that the healthy body rejects and destroys because they have not received good information and therefore have no constructive role to play. When the body is in a weakened state, these neoplastons are not destroyed but rather are left at the mercy of cancer-causing agents that invade the system and "turn them on." They begin to multiply, forming large, constantly growing lumps. They are victims of bad information and assume a destructive role in the body.

This is where antineoplastons come in—as a means of relaying positive messages. Antineoplastons are able to send instructions to abnormal or cancerous cells that can then allow them to differentiate or specialize, thus restoring the body's normal defense mechanisms. The beauty of the treatment is that harmful drugs, radiation, and surgery are not required. The body virtually heals itself.

A Biochemical Defense System

According to the research done by Dr. Burzynski and others in this country as well as abroad, antineoplastons are components of a biochemical defense system that parallels our immune system. Unlike the immune system, which protects us by destroying invading agents or defective cells, this biochemical defense system protects us by reprogramming, or normalizing, defective cells. Errors in cell programming may lead to such diverse disorders as cancer, benign tumors, certain skin diseases, AIDS, and Parkinson's disease.

Evolution of a Therapy

How did Stanislaw Burzynski develop this amazing therapy? The doctor's progress in medical research is characterized by a rare ability to look further, to take that extra step onto an untried path and go beyond the status quo. Considering that the doctor was born into a family with a passion for learning, these traits aren't altogether surprising. His parents had university degrees, his father a total of five before retiring as a university professor. Stanislaw followed suit, becoming at age twenty-five one of Poland's youngest men ever to earn both an M.D. and a Ph.D. He began his research at one of Poland's finest medical schools, the Lublin Medical Academy. Its prestigious faculty provided the mentors he needed to shape his embryonic theories on anticancer defense mechanisms.

The Polish government eventually allowed him to emigrate to the United States, and by 1970 Dr. Burzynski had become a staff member at Baylor College of Medicine, continuing his theories about the causes and treatments of cancer. Because his research had been interrupted by obligatory military service, nearly a decade had passed since he had fixed on the notion that the human body must possess a built-in system to resist cancer and similar diseases. He believed that without this system, no one could hope to ward off the cancer-creating "sea of carcinogens" that surround us. Of course, believing that a natural defense system exists does not explain what it is made up of and how it works, but mentors from his university days offered some clues.

From a former chemistry professor Dr. Burzynski had learned about the information-carrying peptides, which are related to the antineoplastons he had yet to uncover. Other clues had come from Dr. Marian Mazur, professor at the Polish Academy of Science and a widely acclaimed authority in the cybernetic field of science. Cybernetics looks at how systems work; one of its key elements is feedback, which provides a way to control and communicate within a system. If cancer cells become destructive because they have received only bad information, the task is not to kill them but to get the right information to them to make them normal and healthy. Cybernetics provides insight into the nature of improving communications within a system so that the desired information or feedback is properly transmitted. A household thermostat is an example of a feedback device: a tool used to close the gap between an actual result—say, room temperature of 90 degrees—and a desired result—a more comfortable 70 degrees.

Dr. Burzynski concluded that active ingredient of the body's cancer defense system might be found in the family of peptides—small blood proteins—which are known to communicate with and affect the growth of cells. Within that system, these substances could operate as a feedback device to correct the difference between actual cancer cells and the desired healthy cells or to reprogram cancer cells with good information so that they could become constructive and vital instead of pathogenic.

Peptides are a popular subject of modern medical research. Nearly fifty different types have been found that can stimulate cell growth. One, known as peptide T, is attracting attention for its potential in treating AIDS. Dr. Burzynski is thus by no means the only scientist exploring the potency of peptides, but he has been at it longer than most and has achieved findings unique to cancer therapy.

An early discovery involved the level of peptides in advanced cancer patients. Their blood samples revealed only 2 to 3 percent of the amount typically found in healthy bodies—a drastic difference. If peptides, as Dr. Burzynski assumed, played a role in the body's natural defense system, these cancer patients had at some point been disarmed. They were victims of misinformation, because there were not enough peptides to carry good information to the cancer cells.

The next task was to determine exactly what kind of peptides cancerous bodies lack. Burzynski put his doctorate in biochemistry to good use, studying the makeup and structure of the deficient substances and uncovering an interesting effect. When applied to tissue cultures, the peptides missing from cancer patients actually suppressed the growth of human cancer cells.

But while progress was evident, the puzzle was far from solved. It was not enough to know that antineoplastons could carry appropriate information to cancerous cells; it had to be determined how to get them to do it in order to ameliorate tumor growths. Dr. Burzynski turned to his knowledge of systems, cybernetic science, and information theory. The idea of using feedback to adjust and correct an obvious imbalance seemed appropriate to the possible role of antineoplastons in treating cancer.

The Treatment: Reprogramming Cancer Cells

Dr. Burzynski's concept constituted a scientific leap, yet it appears amazingly simple in light of the most basic function peptides perform: They transmit information to the cells. Some aim to spur on, others to inhibit, cellular growth, but they all do it by sending messages the body can obey.

Dr. Burzynski likens the process to the use of the alphabet: "It's like having twenty-six alphabet letters—you can create an infinite variety of words."[428] Using the right "code" becomes the key to reprogramming cancerous cells. Theoretically, it is possible to stop a peptide messenger carrying dangerous, damaging goods and hand over a more beneficent, favorable package for it to deliver instead.

The best time to change the peptide code is when cells are new and immature. Guided by good information, the cells can successfully pass through all the normal stages of development. They can gradually take on the special traits they need to serve different parts of the body—in other words, differentiate. When cells differentiate, they have reached maturity. Imagine being stuck in childhood or puberty, never given the means to change and grow into a finally functioning adult. This is the state of a cancer cell. It doesn't know how to differentiate and mature, because its genetic code is garbled. In a healthy body with a sufficient level of peptides and antineoplastons, good information is quickly communicated to the cancer cell, and the cell is rendered harmless. But when these levels are low, the cancer cell continues to be victimized by the wrong information. Dr. Burzynski's treatment is aimed at ending the cancer cell's confusion. He puts antineoplastons into the bloodstream to carry the proper genetic code, halt the growth of useless tumors, and encourage cancer cells to differentiate.

Antineoplastons are not foreign substances. Because they appear naturally in the body—and evidently are found at a much higher level in healthy bodies—they don't pose a toxic threat. This fact alone sets Dr. Burzynski's approach miles apart from traditional cancer therapies. Radiation treatments and chemotherapy destroy cancer cells but also destroy any other cells in their path.

Two significant observations have been made about the side effects of antineoplaston treatment. First, most patients experience virtually no side effects. The few that have appeared have been minor, short-lived, and easily controlled, such as skin rashes, chills, and fever. The second and more remarkable observation is that the treatment can actually create positive side effects in decided contrast to traditional medical treatments. Patients have shown increases in white and red blood cell counts, decreases in blood cholesterol, and stimulated skin growth; these and other effects are known to aid the body's natural healing powers. Antineoplaston therapy has tremendous promise not just in theory but in practice.

However, a new medicine or medical treatment is not accepted overnight. The medical and scientific communities as well as certain governmental bodies set rigid testing standards to ensure the safety and effectiveness of every supposed curative. Antineoplastons are no exception.

Tests and Results

For several decades Dr. Burzynski has been subjecting his theory to the testing procedure required to prove its worth, and it is holding up well under pressure. More than 60 percent of the patients treated during the Burzynski Research Institute's phase I testing showed considerable improvement, whereas the norm is only 3 percent at best.

Each phase of testing has different goals. Phase I is designed to examine any side effects that may occur and to determine proper dosages of the antineoplaston "medicine." Phase II entails a more specific study of whether and how the medicine acts to reduce or eliminate cancerous growth, and phase III would take an even closer look at these issues, among larger groups of people with the same types of cancer.

When phase I clinical trials began, Dr. Burzynski didn't expect much in the way of an anticancer effect. His aim was to find out how much medicine patients should be given, starting with very small doses that could be increased over time. He had no way of knowing but could only suspect which kinds of cancer would respond best to his treatment. What he expected and what he got were two different things.

The results in the best cases of twenty different phase I trials showed significant anticancer activity. In the most successful trial, not only did more than 60 percent of the patients respond to treatment; more than 20 percent remained cancer-free for over five years. These patients suffered from some of the most serious and difficult-to-treat forms of cancer, including advanced lung and bladder cancer, and malignant mesothelioma—a type of cancer that results from asbestos exposure and is especially resistant to traditional medicine.

In phase II trials, patients are grouped according to their basic type of cancer. Depending on how and where those basic types develop in the body, different phase II treatments are tried. For example, in current trials with breast cancer, treatment varies depending on whether the disease has spread to the lungs or to the liver or bones.

In 1992, twenty-four patients with malignant lymphoma (cancer of the lymphatic system) had been treated in phase II trials. Chemotherapy had failed to help nearly 70 percent of these patients. Only certain forms of this cancer, such as Hodgkin's disease, have ever shown real success from conventional treatment. But with antineoplaston care, 85 percent showed vast improvement.

The most impressive results have been in brain cancers (astrocytoma stages III and IV and glioblastoma) and metastatic cancer of the prostate. In a small phase II trial of astrocytoma conducted by Dr. Burzynski, twenty patients were enrolled. All diagnoses were biopsy-confirmed. All but one patient had received (and failed) one or more prior standard therapies. Four patients achieved complete remission and two others partial remission. The responses of ten patients were classified as objective stabilization (less than 50 percent decrease of tumor size). Since the end of this study in May 1990, some of these patients have achieved partial and even complete remission. Even if they are only preliminary findings, such results are impressive in this type and stage of cancer.

In another phase II study of stage IV prostate cancer refractory to hormonal treatment begun in 1988, two complete and three partial remissions were reported in a group of fourteen patients. Seven patients obtained objective stabilization.

In a 1997 interview, Dr. Burzynski offers us more of the clinic's success stories:

> When we started our program, we concentrated on the type of cancers that are uniformly deadly, such terrible types of malignant tumors as primary malignant brain tumors that are known in medical terminology as astrocytoma, glioblastoma, and medulla blastoma. These tumors are uniformly deadly. Practically everybody who develops high-grade astrocytoma or glioblastoma dies from the disease. There's no cure available, and the death comes quickly, usually within a year.

We concentrated on the treatment of such highly malignant tumors to prove a point that antineoplastons work. Otherwise, if there are some other treatments available, we could be accused of perhaps using these additional treatments which could make the tumors disappear. But those treatments do not exist. If we are able to eliminate highly malignant brain tumors by the use of antineoplastons, these are the first cases in medical history of this happening. Because we concentrate our efforts on the treatment of such bad malignant brain tumors, of course, most of our statistics concentrate on these tumors. We already finished three clinical trials, phase II trials, in such malignant brain tumors. And we found that the success rate of the patients who are responding to the treatment is between 67 to 80 percent among these trials, which means that only 20 percent to 33 percent of the patients do not have any proper response to the treatment.

We already have long-term follow-up for some of these patients, including eight-year follow-up when the tumors disappeared and did not come back. We can say that we were able to not only decrease and eliminate these tumors, but also cure a number of patients from these tumors. We continue to have clinical trials in different types of malignant brain tumors. Currently, we have over twenty different clinical trials in the area of malignant brain tumors, and we are accepting the patients through such trials. If somebody is interested we can, of course, offer him the treatment, and then he can go back home and continue the treatment back home under the care of his doctor.[429]

The Clinic

The Burzynski Clinic in southwest Houston currently sees approximately 70 to 120 patients each month. The clinic operates on an outpatient basis. The average period of care involves an intensive two-to three-week period with patients visiting the clinic daily followed by an additional four to twelve months of self-administered care at home. The average cost of treatment is between $25,000 and $30,000.

The antineoplastons that have been responsible for the dramatic results mentioned above are manufactured in Dr. Burzynski's plant in Stafford, Texas. According to Dr. Burzynski, they are considered a form of chemotherapy because a chemotherapeutic agent is technically any "organized mixture of chemicals that fight a malignancy." However, they do not have the devastating side effects of the traditional class of chemotherapeutic drugs because they are formulations that are identical to proteins that are present in the body. Natural antineoplastons are small proteins isolated from human urine or blood. Synthetic antineoplastons are chemically identical to the natural proteins but are synthetically derived. Synthetics are easier and cheaper to manufacture and are even more efficacious in treating specific cancers such as brain and prostate cancer. Other cancers, though, respond better to the natural substances.

Dr. Burzynski uses a deliberately coordinated assortment of antineoplastons, both synthetic and natural, as the case requires. When he thinks it is appropriate, he refers patients for other types of treatment (chemotherapy, radiation, or surgery) to augment the antineoplaston injection or capsule therapy. While he has had little success with cancer of the testicles and childhood leukemia, he has had astounding results with brain tumors, malignant lymphomas, and cancer of the bladder and prostate.

The Burzynski clinic's latest report from January 2012 shows that out of 1,849 patients treated for the fifteen most common cancer types treated at the clinic, the average objective response (percentage of individuals whose cancer has measurably improved) was at 50 percent. For some cancers, including ovarian and non-Hodgkin's lymphoma, the objective response exceeded 60 percent. In all but three of the fifteen most commonly treated cancers, a greater percentage of patients experienced stable disease (where the condition is not decreasing or increasing in extent or severity) than progressive disease (where the condition worsens).

Looking to the Future

There are currently ten FDA-sponsored clinical trials underway to assess the antineoplaston treatment in treating patients with various forms of cancer. As of January 2012, there is one open clinical trial.

The possibilities of Dr. Burzynski's therapy appear endless. Antineoplastons correct (i.e., stop) cancer development in a way the body understands and easily tolerates. Even with phase I treatments, which aren't intended to produce maximum benefits, some patients emerged cancer-free. Of course, successful outcomes result from traditional approaches as well. Careful surgery can aid recovery, and chemotherapy has had particular success with rarer types of cancer such as Hodgkin's disease and childhood leukemia.

What Dr. Burzynski offers is an opportunity to use and strengthen the body's natural defense system. The need to explore and develop antineoplastons and other safe remedies will continue as long as people are exposed to air pollution, radiation, chemicals, ultraviolet rays, and the like. For more information on this therapy, contact:

Burzynski Clinic
9432 Katy Freeway
Houston, Texas 77055
(800) 714-7181
www.burzynskiclinic.com

Dr. Burzynski and his colleagues routinely publish the results of their latest research; recent study results may be found at the following website: http://www.burzynskiclinic.com/scientific-publications.html

DR. NICHOLAS GONZALEZ'S ENZYME THERAPY

For more than two decades, Nicholas Gonzalez, M.D., has refined an unconventional and promising cancer therapy that involves patient-specific dietary changes, detoxification techniques, and the use of supplements with a particular emphasis on pancreatic enzymes. Early in his medical school studies, Gonzalez had the rare opportunity to meet a true visionary, Dr. William Donald Kelley, who had recently been in the news because of his alternative cancer treatment of actor Steve McQueen. Although an orthodontist rather than a medical doctor, Kelley had been a trailblazer in the field of cancer medicine by curing himself of pancreatic cancer in the early 1960s. Through connections with the head of Memorial Sloan-Kettering Cancer Center, Gonzalez was able to devise a means to evaluate Kelley's work, which involved interviewing over 1,000 of Kelley's patients. Gonzalez' research ultimately led him to embrace Kelley's cancer therapy and change his entire focus to become an alternative oncologist.

According to Gonzalez:

Most conventional cancer researchers propose that the disease develops from normal cells in any of our various tissues, the end result of defects in the DNA occurring spontaneously due to exposure to environmental toxins or as part of the normal aging process. . . . Dr. Kelley believes, however, that cancer forms only from stem cells, undifferentiated precursors located in all our various tissues, that serve as replacements for those cells lost due to normal turnover, disease, injury, or aging. . . . Kelley does agree with mainstream scientists that small numbers of cancer cells form in all of us each day, but only rarely do these mutants take hold and lead to clinical disease. Conventional researchers argue that the immune system, especially the natural killer cells, protect us from such malignancies. But Dr. Kelley disagrees: He claims certain pancreatic enzymes, particularly the proteolytic or protein-digesting enzymes—and not the immune system—represent the first line of defense against malignancy.[430]

Building on the research of his mentor, William Donald Kelley, D.D.S., Gonzalez treats his patients with enzymes derived from pig pancreas. The substance contains a type of proteolytic, or protein-degrading, enzyme that is useful in digesting the protein coating of cancer cells. This is important because it is a necessary step before the cancer cells are destroyed by the body's immune cells. In addition, pancreatic enzymes can stimulate anticancer factors in the blood, that is, natural killer cells, T-cells, and tumor necrosis factor.

Success Rate

In 1994, Gonzalez began a study on enzyme therapy in the treatment of patients with inoperable adenocarcinoma of the pancreas. Published in 1999 in the journal *Nutrition and Cancer*, the study showed a significantly higher survival rate among those patients who underwent enzyme therapy. Out of the eleven patients observed in the study, nine survived one year, five lived for two years, four made it to three years, and two survived beyond four years. Pancreatic cancer is one of the most untreatable and quickly fatal cancers than befall us, so Gonzalez' results were quite remarkable. Having been told that a positive result for his study would have been for 3 out of 10 patients with stage IV pancreatic cancer to survive one year, Gonzalez surpassed this goal by a considerable amount. In contrast, a trial evaluating 126 patients treated for pancreatic cancer with the conventional cancer drug gemcitabine showed that not one person survived beyond nineteen months.

A 2007 article by Dr. Gonzalez and Linda Isaacs, M.D., that was published in the peer-reviewed journal *Alternative Therapies* provided the case studies of thirty-six patients treated with enzyme therapy. Despite being given a poor prognosis and having advanced cancer, each of these patients experienced extraordinary survival rates.[431]

Treatment Specifics

Patients are instructed to take up to 45 g of the pancreatic enzyme product daily through oral doses. Several other individualized nutritional protocols are implemented that include following a specialized diet (which can range from almost entirely vegetarian to a more meat-based regimen), and taking a variety of supplements containing vitamins, minerals, and other food concentrates. The use of coffee enemas and other detoxifying tools are also utilized during treatment.

Every patient seen at the clinic is evaluated during two in-depth sessions. The total cost of these sessions is $4,000. The supplements prescribed to patients are sold by an independent manufacturer and cost, on average, $800 a month. The cost of a six-month follow up visit is $850, and routine office visits run $250. At any given time, Dr. Gonzalez and his colleagues treat approximately 400 cancer patients at their Manhattan office.

For more information on this therapy, contact

Nicholas J. Gonzalez, M.D., P.C.
36A East 36th Street, Suite 204
New York, NY 10016
(212) 213-3337
http://www.dr-gonzalez.com/index.htm

REVICI THERAPY

The late biochemist and physician Dr. Emmanuel Revici was the innovator of a remarkable nontoxic form of chemotherapy that has effectively treated different forms of cancer and other illnesses. During the first part of his long career, which began in the 1920s, Dr. Revici conducted groundbreaking research into the role of lipids, which are fundamental building blocks of human biology, in the development of cancer. Much of Dr. Revici's studies centered on the observation that lipids are insoluble in blood and therefore selectively absorbed by damaged body tissue. His research also determined that tumors have a high concentration of abnormal free lipids.

Using this information, Dr. Revici devised a method in which natural substances derived from plant, mineral, and animal material could be integrated with lipids to create a special compound. By introducing these compounds to the bloodstream, the treatment transports therapeutic agents to diseased and abnormal tissue where they help restore normal body function. In treating cancer patients, Revici utilized selenium compounds due to their exceptional capacity to be absorbed by tumors and subsequently destroy cancer cells and shrink the size of tumors.

Treatment Success

Revici Medical, the New York-based nonprofit dedicated to advancing the work of Dr. Revici, reports that the therapy has compiled numerous case studies that detail significant improvement in the condition of patients with prostate, kidney, breast, pancreatic, and other cancers. In some cases, a full clinical remission has been reported. Because the substances added to these lipid compounds are natural and nontoxic, the majority of patients taking Revici's medications experience no significant adverse reactions.

Raphael Kellman, M.D., practices an integrative cancer treatment that incorporates the principles of the Revici Therapy. The therapy aims to improve the function of cell, organ, and systems through natural medicine and technologies designed to improve oxygenation and restore homeostasis. For more information on this therapy, contact:

> Raphael Kellman, M.D.
> 150 East 55th Street, 6th Floor
> New York, NY 10022
> (212) 717-1118
> http://raphaelkellmanmd.com/

ADDITIONAL THERAPIES

Ozone Therapy

Not to be confused with atmospheric ozone, medical ozone is pure and concentrated, and has unique healing properties. Although ozone therapy is not widely practiced in the United States, Europeans and Cubans have been benefiting from these treatments for years.

Ozone is used both prophylactically and as a treatment for a wide variety of diseases, including cancer. An antineoplastic substance (one that inhibits the growth of tumors), ozone stimulates the production of white blood cells and increases production of alpha interferon, interleukin-2, and tumor necrosis factor. It has also been found to enhance the action of various antitumor drugs.

According to the naturopathic physician Dr. Stanley Beyerle, prostate cancer patients often respond quite well to ozone treatment if the cancer is left encapsulated (that is, not biopsied). Other types of cancer that Beyerle has seen major improvements with, using ozone, are tonsillar, throat, ovarian, colon, and breast cancer.[432]

One mode of delivery of medical ozone is autohemotherapy, in which a portion of the patient's blood is mixed, outside the body, with a dose of ozone/oxygen, and then reintroduced into the circulation. Other methods used are rectal insufflations and drinking ozonated water.

Individualized Vaccines

When some of a patient's own cancer cells are combined in a laboratory with some of his or her white blood cells, it's possible—in some cases—to create a personalized vaccine that works to stimulate the patient's immune system to destroy the cancer. Dramatic results using this approach have been seen in Europe and in clinics following Dr. Josef Issels's immunotherapy treatment.

Coley's Toxins

This is another, older, vaccine approach to cancer. Dr. William Coley, who practiced in the early part of the 20th century, found that certain inactivated bacteria could be given to patients to energize their immune systems against cancer. It was as if, by first fighting against the weaker opponent, the bacteria, the body built up its defenses and became more able to fight the cancer. Research has shown this treatment to be of significant value, although a perceived drawback is the fever that develops shortly after the vaccine is given. This, according to proponents of Coley's treatment, is actually a sign that the vaccine is working, and should not be suppressed.

714-X

Based on the work of Dr. Gaston Naessens, 714X is a compound made from nitrogen-rich camphor and organic salts, which is given to render the immune system more efficient in its battle against cancer cells. Naessens's theory, which grew from extensive cancer research using a high-powered microscope that he developed, is based on the observation that cancer cells cannibalize the body to feed their need for nitrogen. By supplying nitrogen to cancer cells via 714-X, the growth of cancer can be stymied while the body's own natural defenses are fortified. Naessens achieved impressive results curing cancer in his native France and his adopted country of Canada, and 714-X continues to be made available through Cerbe, Inc. Results of 714-X treatment, which usually consists of a series of injections into the lymph nodes of the groin, include tumor shrinkage, weight gain, a lessening of pain, and extended survival time. People receiving this treatment are cautioned not to take vitamins E or B12 while they undergo treatment, as it may counter the effects.

Hydrazine Sulfate

This experimental treatment shows promise, as it helps cancer patients regain lost weight. It seems to improve appetite and feelings of well-being and may help shrink tumors.[433, 434]

Thymus Extract

The thymus is responsible for a number of immune system functions, including the important production of T lymphocytes, which are a kind of white blood cell that controls "cell-mediated immunity." This simply refers to the immune mechanisms not controlled by antibodies. Cell-mediated immunity is vital in warding off infection by specific bacteria, yeast (including *Candida albicans*), fungi, parasites, and viruses (including herpes simplex, Epstein-Barr, and the viruses that cause hepatitis). Furthermore, cell-mediated immunity is essential for strengthening the system so that it can fight against the development of cancer.

Ukrain

The plant celandine is combined with thiophosphoric acid to create ukrain, a substance used by so-called terminal cancer patients to block tumor growth and rev up their immune system.

Carnivora

A treatment for skin cancer, carnivora is a mixture of the juice of the Venus flytrap, alcohol, and purified water. This preparation, applied topically, stimulates T-helper cells.

Iscador

This is a mistletoe derivative given by injection. Iscador has been shown effective in the treatment of breast, cervical, bladder, bronchial, ovarian, and skin cancers.[435, 436]

Larch Arabinogalactan

This is a substance derived from the Western larch tree. It's used in the form of a powder called Larix, or Ara-6, which stimulates immune cell activity and raises patients' energy levels.

The most important piece of knowledge when preventing and fighting cancer is this: You have control. While toxins exist in our environments, foods, workplaces, and other consumer goods, we each have the ability to take power over our own choices. With the protocols I have laid out for eating, exercising, and avoiding toxins, you have all the tools to make healthy, effective, and natural choices to eliminate cancer.

Gary Null's Healthy and Delicious Anticancer Recipes

The following recipes coincide with my recommendations for healthy eating—namely, these meals aim to include those foods which actively fight cancer, and exclude those foods which have been shown to be carcinogenic.

Appetizers

BARLEY WITH COLLARD GREENS AND LEEKS

1 cup collard greens, sliced thin

¼ cup vegetable broth

½ cup leeks, sliced

2 cloves garlic, minced

1 cup fresh tomatoes, chopped

¾ cup mushrooms, sliced (reserve a few slices for garnish)

½ cup red bell peppers, sliced

¼ cup fresh parsley, chopped

½ teaspoon dried oregano

Sea salt to taste

½ teaspoon freshly ground black pepper
3 cups barley, cooked

Place the collard greens in a steamer and steam over boiling water for 20 minutes.

Heat the vegetable broth in a skillet and sauté the leeks and garlic for about 3 minutes until tender.

Add the tomatoes, mushrooms, bell pepper, parsley, oregano, salt, and black pepper, and sauté for about 10 minutes, stirring frequently.

Add the steamed collard greens and sauté for an additional 5 minutes.

Garnish with sliced mushrooms and serve with cooked barley.

Yield: 2 servings

BAVARIAN CABBAGE
¼ cup vegetable broth
1 small yellow onion, diced
1 clove garlic, chopped
1 oz. kombu or arame seaweed, soaked in water for about 10 minutes to reconstitute
1 cup green cabbage, shredded
½ cup red cabbage, shredded
1 Granny Smith apple, diced
1 teaspoon maple syrup
Sea salt to taste
½ teaspoon freshly ground black pepper
1 tablespoon apple cider vinegar

Heat the vegetable broth in a large pan and sauté the onion, garlic, and seaweed until tender, about 3 minutes.

Add green and red cabbage, apple, maple syrup, salt, pepper, and vinegar, and cook, covered, over low heat for approximately 20 minutes.
Garnish with fresh fruit.

Yield: 2 servings

EGGPLANT CAPONATA
½ cup vegetable broth
1 large yellow onion, diced
2 cloves garlic, minced
2 stalks celery, sliced
4 tomatoes, chopped
½ cup fresh basil, chopped
2 small eggplants, diced
4 tablespoons pine nuts
2 tablespoons capers, drained
2 tablespoons apple cider vinegar
Sea salt to taste
½ teaspoon freshly ground black pepper

Heat the vegetable broth in a skillet and sauté the onion, garlic, and celery until the onion is translucent.
Add the tomatoes and basil and simmer, covered, for 10 minutes, stirring frequently.
Add the eggplant, pine nuts, capers, vinegar, salt, and pepper, and simmer for 15 minutes.
Serve with toasted bread.

Yields: 4 servings

CREAMY TOFU DIP
2 cups silken tofu
2 tablespoons chopped fresh parsley

2 tablespoons prepared mustard
2 tablespoons apple cider vinegar
2 tablespoons chopped fresh dill (reserve some for garnish)
Sea salt to taste
½ teaspoon freshly ground black pepper
¼ cup chives, chopped

Place the tofu, parsley, mustard, vinegar, dill, salt, pepper, and chives in a food processor or blender and purée until smooth.
Place in a serving dish and garnish with dill.
Serve chilled, with raw vegetables.

Yield: 6 servings

DATE SPREAD
1 cup cooked red kidney beans
2 tablespoons dates, chopped
1 tablespoon fresh mint, chopped
½ cup cashews, chopped
1 tablespoon chia seeds
2 tablespoons grade B maple syrup
1 teaspoon almond extract
1 teaspoon vanilla extract
Sea salt to taste

Purée the beans, dates, and mint in a food processor until smooth.
Add the cashews, chia seeds, maple syrup, almond extract, vanilla extract, and salt, and pulse until well mixed.
Serve with crackers or raw vegetables.

Yield: 5 servings

HOLIDAY STUFFED MUSHROOMS
6 large mushrooms, de-stemmed (mince stems and set aside)
2 tablespoons extra virgin olive oil

1 medium yellow onion, diced

2 cloves garlic, minced

1 red bell pepper, chopped

2 tablespoons flax seed, ground

2 teaspoons fresh parsley, chopped

½ teaspoon fresh sage, chopped

½ teaspoon fresh rosemary, chopped

½ teaspoon fresh thyme

Sea salt to taste

½ teaspoon freshly ground black pepper

1 tablespoon fresh chives, chopped, for garnish

Preheat oven to 350° F.

Place the mushroom caps on a baking sheet sprayed with nonstick olive oil and bake for 15 minutes, or until brown.

Heat olive oil in a skillet and sauté onion, garlic, and red pepper until the onion is translucent.

Place the minced mushroom stems, onion, garlic, red pepper, flaxseed, parsley, sage, rosemary, thyme, salt, and pepper in a food processor and pulse until coarsely chopped.

Stuff mushroom caps with filling and garnish with chives.

Yield: 6 servings

SPICY TOMATO SALSA

1 cup fresh tomatoes, chopped

¼ cup red onion, chopped

1 tablespoon fresh parsley, chopped

4 tablespoons fresh basil, chopped

1 teaspoon ginger, chopped

1 teaspoon extra-virgin olive oil

2 tablespoons fresh hot peppers, minced

Sea salt to taste

½ teaspoon freshly ground black pepper

Combine all the ingredients in a medium bowl and mix until well blended.

Serve with vegetable chips or raw vegetables.

Yield: 6 servings

SPICY BULGUR SALAD

Dressing:
2 tablespoons walnut oil
1 tablespoon raw, unfiltered apple cider vinegar
1 clove garlic, pressed
Sea salt to taste
½ teaspoon freshly ground black pepper
Pinch of cayenne
1 cup bulgur, cooked
1 cup spinach, coarsely chopped
1 jar marinated artichoke hearts, quartered
1 tablespoon fresh basil, chopped
½ teaspoon curry powder
½ cup alfalfa sprouts for garnish

Whisk vinegar, oil, garlic, salt, and pepper together in a small bowl.
Place bulgur, spinach artichoke hearts, basil, and curry powder in a salad bowl and toss the salad with the dressing.
Garnish with alfalfa sprouts.

Yield: 2 servings

Breakfast

AMARANTH PEACH DELIGHT
2 cups water
1 cup amaranth
1 teaspoon chia seeds

½ cup dried peaches, chopped

¼ cup raisins

½ cup pecans, chopped

½ teaspoon ground cinnamon

¼ teaspoon ground cloves

¼ teaspoon ground nutmeg

Combine water, amaranth, and chia seeds in a medium saucepan and bring to a slow boil over medium heat.

After 15 minutes, add the dried peaches, raisins, pecans, cinnamon, cloves, and nutmeg, and cook to desired consistency.

Garnish with pecans.

Yield: 2 servings

BLUEBERRY-APRICOT OATMEAL

1 cup water

¾ cup steel-cut oats

1 tablespoon chia seeds

1 teaspoon ground cinnamon

½ teaspoon ground ginger

½ cup fresh blueberries

½ cup sliced apricot

½ banana, sliced

Bring water to a boil in a medium saucepan, add the steel-cut oats, chia seeds, cinnamon, ginger, blueberries, and apricot slices and reduce heat.

Simmer 5 to 8 minutes to desired consistency, stirring frequently.

Garnish with sliced banana and berries.

Yield: 2 servings

HAWAIIAN RICE CEREAL

¼ cup shredded unsweetened coconut, for garnish
½ cup chopped macadamia nuts
½ cup apple or other fresh juice
1 banana, sliced
½ cup pitted fresh cherries, chopped
½ cup fresh pineapple, chopped
2 cups cooked brown rice
1 teaspoon flax seeds, raw or toasted

Preheat oven to 375° F.
Place unsweetened coconut and macadamia nuts on an ungreased baking pan and bake for 3 to 5 minutes or until light brown.
In a medium saucepan combine the apple juice, banana, cherries, and pineapple and cook over low heat for 3 to 5 minutes.
Stir in the brown rice, flax seeds, and macadamia nuts and cook for an additional 2 minutes.
Garnish with toasted coconut.

Yield: 2 servings

BANANA COCONUT BUCKWHEAT CEREAL

½ cup uncooked cream of buckwheat cereal
¼ cup flaxseed meal
2 ½ cups water
1 tablespoon dried apricot
1 tablespoon dried currants
1 tablespoon raisins
1 ½ teaspoons ground cinnamon
½ cup banana, sliced
¼ cup toasted coconut flakes

Combine cream of buckwheat, flaxseed meal, and water in a medium saucepan and bring to a slow boil over medium heat.

Add the apricots, currants, raisins, and cinnamon, and cook 5 to 8 minutes to desired consistency, stirring frequently.
Garnish with sliced banana and coconut.

Yield: 2 servings

COCONUT NUT RICE
1 cup brown rice, cooked
½ cup toasted coconut flakes (save half for garnish)
½ cup cashews, chopped
½ cup dried apricots, chopped
1 teaspoon chia seeds
1 teaspoon ground cinnamon
½ teaspoon ground nutmeg
¼ cup all-natural apple juice
¼ cup sunflower seeds, for garnish

Combine brown rice with coconut, cashews, apricots, chia seeds, cinnamon, and nutmeg in a medium bowl.
Place half the mixture and the apple juice in a food processor and pulse until coarsely ground.
Add back to the rest of the rice and mix well.
Garnish with apricot pieces and coconut.

Yield: 2 servings

Soups

MISO TOFU SOUP
1 tablespoon walnut oil
4 scallions, sliced
2 cloves garlic, minced
1 large celery stalk, sliced
4 cups water
1 package firm tofu, diced

½ red bell pepper, chopped
½ yellow bell pepper, chopped
3 tablespoons fresh parsley, chopped (save half for garnish)
½ teaspoon oregano
Sea salt to taste
½ teaspoon freshly ground black pepper
4 tablespoons brown rice miso

Heat the oil in a large saucepan and sauté the scallions, garlic, and celery until tender, about 2 minutes.

Add the water, tofu, red and yellow bell pepper, parsley, oregano, salt, and pepper, and simmer for 10 minutes.

Remove 1 cup of hot liquid, dissolve the miso in it, return it to the saucepan, and blend well.

Garnish with parsley.

Yield: 2 servings

PORTUGUESE KALE POTATO SOUP
1 tablespoon olive oil
1 yellow onion, diced
3 cloves garlic, minced
4 cups water
2 cups fresh kale, chopped (reserve 1 tablespoon for garnish)
1 large Yukon gold potato, peeled and cut into cubes
Sea salt to taste
Freshly ground black pepper to taste
Pinch of nutmeg
3 teaspoons spearmint leaves
1 teaspoon paprika, for garnish

Heat the oil in a large saucepan and sauté the onion and garlic until the onion is translucent.

Add the water, kale, potato, salt, pepper, nutmeg, and spearmint, and cook over medium heat for 15 minutes.

Remove the potato from the soup and place in a blender or food processor with some of the cooking liquid and purée until smooth.

Return the puréed potato to the soup and stir until well blended. Garnish with chopped kale and paprika.

Yield: 2 servings

TURNIP AND BLACK BEAN SOUP

1 tablespoon olive oil

1 yellow onion, diced

2 cloves garlic, minced

2 cups black beans, cooked

4 cups water

1 large turnip, diced

Kernels from 1 ear of fresh corn

1 teaspoon fresh thyme, chopped

½ teaspoon cumin

1 bay leaf

Sea salt to taste

½ teaspoon freshly ground black pepper

¼ teaspoon cayenne

2 tablespoons chives, minced, for garnish

Heat the oil in a large saucepan and sauté the onion and garlic until the onion is translucent.

Add the remaining ingredients and simmer over low heat for 20 minutes.

Garnish with chives.

Yield: 4 servings

ALGERIAN CHILI

1 tablespoon olive oil

1 medium yellow onion, diced

4 cloves garlic, minced

2 scallions, chopped (reserve 1 tablespoon for garnish)

1 stalk celery, chopped

4 cups water or vegetable broth

1 tomato, coarsely chopped

1 small dried red chili

1 red bell pepper, chopped

½ tablespoon sweet paprika

1 tablespoon curry powder

½ cup tomato paste

2 teaspoons ground cumin

3 cups navy beans, cooked

1 bay leaf

Pinch of cayenne

3 tablespoons fresh parsley, chopped (reserve 1 tablespoon for garnish)

Sea salt to taste

½ teaspoon freshly ground black pepper

Heat the oil in a large saucepan and sauté the onion, garlic, scallions, and celery until the onion is translucent.

Add the water, tomato, chili pepper, red bell pepper, paprika, curry powder, tomato paste, and cumin, and simmer until the mixture thickens, stirring frequently.

Add the beans, bay leaf, cayenne, parsley, salt, and pepper, and simmer for 15 minutes.

Garnish with parsley and scallions.

Yield: 4 servings

ITALIAN-STYLE PINTO BEAN SOUP

2 tablespoons olive oil

1 yellow onion, diced

2 cloves garlic, minced

1 stalk celery, chopped

1 red bell pepper, chopped

4 cups water

2 cups pinto beans, cooked

2 carrots, sliced

1 cup mushrooms, sliced

½ cup arugula, chopped

½ teaspoon cumin

Sea salt to taste

½ teaspoon freshly ground black pepper

Heat the oil in a large saucepan and sauté the onion, garlic, celery, and red pepper until the onion is translucent.

Add water, beans, carrots, mushrooms, arugula, cumin, salt, and pepper, and simmer over medium heat for 20 minutes.

Yield: 4 servings

FAVORITE VEGETABLE SOUP

2 tablespoons walnut oil

1 yellow onion, diced

2 cloves garlic, diced

1 stalk celery, sliced (reserve a few slices for garnish)

4 cups vegetable stock

1 cup mung beans, cooked

½ red cabbage, sliced

1 tablespoon chopped fresh parsley

½ teaspoon ground oregano

2 tablespoons fresh basil, chopped

1 tablespoon fresh thyme, chopped
Sea salt to taste
½ teaspoon freshly ground black pepper
1 sprig thyme for garnish
1 cup basmati or brown rice, cooked

Heat the oil in a large saucepan and sauté the onion, garlic, and celery until the onion is translucent.

Add vegetable broth, mung beans, cabbage, parsley, oregano, basil, thyme, salt, and pepper, and cook over medium heat for 15 minutes.

Place soup contents in a blender or food processor and purée.

Return the purée to the saucepan and cook until thoroughly heated.

Garnish with celery, rice, and thyme.

Yield: 4 servings

Entrees

APPLE, WALNUT, AND TOFU SALAD

Dressing:

2 tablespoons walnut oil
1 tablespoon lemon juice
1 clove garlic, pressed
Sea salt to taste
½ teaspoon freshly ground black pepper
Pinch cayenne

Salad:

½ cup yellow onion, diced
1 stalk celery, sliced
¼ teaspoon ground cumin

1 Granny Smith apple, diced
1 package firm tofu, diced
½ cup walnuts
½ cup chives

Whisk oil, lemon juice, garlic, salt, pepper, and cayenne together in a small bowl.
Place onion, celery, cumin, apple, tofu, and walnuts in a salad bowl and toss with the dressing.
Garnish with chives.

Yield: 2 servings

BROCCOLI CAULIFLOWER WITH SHIITAKE MUSHROOMS
¾ cup unsweetened almond milk
1 tablespoon oat flour
1 tablespoon flaxseed meal
1 tablespoon grated lemon zest
1 clove garlic, minced
1 scallion, chopped
1 tablespoon fresh oregano, chopped
1 tablespoon fresh thyme, chopped
1 tablespoon fresh basil, chopped
Sea salt to taste
½ teaspoon freshly ground black pepper
¼ teaspoon cayenne
1 head broccoli, separated into florets
½ head cauliflower, separated into florets
½ cup shiitake mushrooms, chopped
1 cup extra-firm tofu, diced
½ red bell pepper, chopped
½ cup grated vegan cheese

Preheat oven to 325° F.

Whisk together almond milk, flour, flaxseed meal, lemon zest, garlic, scallions, oregano, thyme, basil, salt, pepper, and cayenne in a small bowl.

Combine the broccoli, cauliflower, mushrooms, tofu, and red pepper in a mixing bowl.

Lightly grease a baking dish with olive oil, and add the broccoli mixture.

Pour the almond milk sauce evenly over the vegetables.

Sprinkle with vegan cheese and bake until the sauce thickens, approximately 25 minutes.

Yields: 2 to 4 servings

BROWN RICE WITH PEPPERS AND HERBS

1 tablespoon walnut oil
1 medium yellow onion, chopped
2 cloves garlic, minced
½ red bell pepper, diced
½ yellow bell pepper, diced
½ bell pepper, diced
1½ cups brown rice, cooked
¾ tablespoon fresh parsley, chopped
½ teaspoon fresh tarragon, chopped
Sea salt to taste
Freshly ground black pepper to taste
¼ cup arugula
½ cup cherry tomatoes

Heat the oil in a large saucepan and sauté the onion and garlic until the onion is translucent.

Add the peppers and sauté for a minute or two.

Add the rice, parsley, tarragon, salt, and pepper and sauté for 3 to 5 minutes.

Garnish with arugula and sliced cherry tomatoes.

Yield: 2 servings

CAULIFLOWER WITH GARLIC HUMMUS SAUCE

1 cup chickpeas, cooked

3 tablespoons tahini

2 cloves garlic, minced

1 teaspoon lemon juice

Sea salt to taste

½ teaspoon freshly ground pepper

¼ teaspoon cayenne

1 cup cauliflower florets

1 cup red bell pepper, chopped

1 small red onion, diced

3 tablespoons fresh parsley, chopped (reserve 1 tablespoon for garnish)

¼ teaspoon turmeric

½ cup unsalted whole cashews

2 cups rice, cooked

Preheat oven to 425° F.

Place chickpeas, tahini, garlic, lemon juice, salt, pepper, and cayenne in a food processor and purée until smooth.

In a mixing bowl, combine the chickpea purée, cauliflower, red pepper, red onion, parsley, turmeric, and cashews and mix well.

Pour the mixture into a lightly-greased, 9-inch by 12-inch baking dish and cover with foil.

Bake for 15 to 20 minutes, or until the cauliflower is tender.

Serve over rice.

Garnish with parsley.

Yields: 2 servings

BRUSSELS SPROUTS CREOLE

2 tablespoons olive oil
1 large yellow onion, diced
2 garlic cloves, minced
½ red bell pepper, chopped
½ orange bell pepper, chopped
1 fresh tomato, chopped
½ cup water
2 tablespoons fresh basil, chopped
2 tablespoons fresh parsley, chopped
¼ cup olives, pitted and sliced
1 tablespoon grated lemon zest
Sea salt to taste
½ teaspoon freshly ground black pepper
2 cups Brussels sprouts, steamed
½ head red leaf lettuce

Heat the oil in a medium saucepan and sauté the onion, garlic, and bell peppers until the onion is translucent.
Add the tomato, water, basil, parsley, olives, lemon zest, salt, and pepper and let simmer for 15 minutes, stirring occasionally.
Add the Brussels sprouts and simmer for a few minutes until warm.
Serve on a bed of red leaf lettuce.

Yield: 4 to 6 servings

BUTTERNUT SQUASH WITH TOASTED SESAME SAUCE

1 butternut squash, cut into ½-inch pieces
1 tablespoon toasted sesame oil
3 tablespoons tahini
1 clove garlic, minced
1 tablespoon fresh parsley, chopped

Sea salt to taste
½ teaspoon freshly ground pepper
2 tablespoons gomasio
¼ cup sesame seeds
½ cup baby mesclun

Steam the squash for 15 to 20 minutes until tender.
Remove from the heat and place in individual dishes.
Whisk together the oil, tahini, garlic, parsley, salt, and pepper in a small bowl.
Pour the tahini mixture over the steamed squash.
Sprinkle with gomasio, parsley, and sesame seeds.
Garnish with baby mesclun

Yield: 2 to 3 servings

CHICKPEA AND ZUCCHINI CURRY
2 tablespoons olive oil
1 large yellow onion, sliced
4 cloves garlic, minced
1 teaspoon mustard seeds
1 large tomato, chopped
1 can tomato paste
½ cup water
1 tablespoon tamari
2 thin slices of fresh ginger root, minced
2 teaspoons turmeric
¼ teaspoon cayenne pepper
2 teaspoons ground cumin
2 teaspoons ground coriander
1 teaspoon ground cinnamon
½ teaspoon ground cloves
Sea salt to taste

½ teaspoon freshly ground black pepper

1 cup chickpeas, cooked

2 medium zucchini, sliced

4 to 5 cups cooked brown rice

2 tablespoons fresh chives, chopped

Heat the oil in a large skillet and sauté the onion and garlic until the onion is translucent.

Add the mustard seeds and cook until they pop, stirring frequently.

Add the tomato, tomato paste, water, tamari, ginger, turmeric, cayenne, cumin, coriander, cinnamon, cloves, salt, pepper, and chickpeas and stir well.

Cover and simmer for about 15 minutes, stirring frequently.

Add the zucchini, mix well, and let simmer for another 10 minutes.

Serve with brown rice.

Garnish with chives.

Yield: 4 to 6 servings

CRUNCHY HERBED GREEN BEANS

2 tablespoons olive oil

1 small yellow onion, diced

2 cloves garlic, minced

¼ cup water

1 pound green beans, trimmed

½ cup green pepper

½ cup red pepper

½ cup yellow pepper

½ teaspoon marjoram

1 tablespoon fresh rosemary, chopped

Sea salt to taste

½ teaspoon freshly ground black pepper

Heat the oil in a skillet and sauté the onion, garlic and peppers until the onions are translucent.

Add the water, green beans, marjoram, rosemary, salt, and pepper and sauté for 3 to 4 minutes, until the green beans are just tender.

Yield: 4 servings

GOULASH

1 tablespoon olive oil
1 medium yellow onion, chopped
2 shallots, minced
2 cloves garlic, minced
1 stalk celery, chopped
1 large tomato, chopped
1 cup vegetable broth
1 package firm tofu, diced
1 cup asparagus, sliced
½ cup chickpeas, cooked
¼ teaspoon caraway seeds
½ teaspoon Hungarian paprika
Sea salt to taste
½ teaspoon freshly ground black pepper
1 tablespoon Bragg's Liquid Aminos
¼ cup tahini

Heat the oil in a large saucepan and sauté the onion, shallots, garlic, and celery until the onion is translucent.

Add tomato and vegetable broth and simmer for 15 minutes.

Add tofu, asparagus, chickpeas, caraway seeds, paprika, salt, and pepper, and simmer for 10 minutes.

Add the Bragg's Liquid Aminos and stir well.

Serve with tahini.

Yield: 4 servings

GREEN PEA MILLET COUSCOUS

2 tablespoons walnut oil

2 shallots, minced

2 cloves garlic, minced

1½ cups vegetable broth

¾ cup millet

1 tablespoon chia seeds

½ cup fresh peas

⅓ cup fresh spearmint, chopped

1 tablespoon Bragg's Liquid Aminos, or to taste

½ cup parsley leaves

½ teaspoon paprika

Heat the oil in a large saucepan and sauté the shallots and garlic for 3 minutes, until tender.

Add the vegetable broth, millet, chia seeds, peas, and spearmint and simmer over low heat for about 15 to 20 minutes, or until water is absorbed and millet is tender.

Remove from heat and stir in Bragg's Liquid Aminos.

Garnish with parsley and paprika.

Yield: 2 servings

PURPLE CABBAGE AND SPAGHETTI SQUASH STIR-FRY

1 tablespoon olive oil

2 scallions, sliced

3 cloves garlic, minced

2 cups vegetable broth

½ spaghetti squash, diced

2 cups broccoli florets

2 cups purple cabbage, sliced

1 package firm tofu, cubed

1 teaspoon fresh ginger, minced

2 tablespoons fresh parsley, chopped

1 tablespoon fresh thyme, chopped

2 tablespoon tamari

½ teaspoon freshly ground black pepper

¼ cup sesame seeds for garnish

Heat the oil in a large saucepan and sauté the scallions and garlic until tender.

Add the vegetable broth, squash, broccoli, cabbage, tofu, ginger, parsley, thyme, tamari, and pepper, and simmer for 15 to 20 minutes until vegetables are tender.

Garnish with the sesame seeds.

Yield: 3 servings

Desserts

BANANA CARAMEL CUSTARD

1 cup almond milk

2 tablespoons arrowroot

2 teaspoons vanilla extract

½ teaspoon almond extract

2 teaspoons ground cinnamon

1 teaspoon ground ginger

½ teaspoon ground nutmeg

1 cup banana, sliced

1 cup maple sugar

1 tablespoon water

In a medium bowl, combine the milk, arrowroot, vanilla extract, almond extract, cinnamon, ginger, and nutmeg and mix well.

Place the mixture in a saucepan over medium heat and simmer, stirring constantly with a whisk or wooden spoon, until thickened. Once thickened, remove from heat and stir in banana slices.

In a small pan over low flame, combine the maple sugar and water and cook until golden brown.

Pour the sugar mixture evenly into a large, greased ramekin (or 4 individual ramekins).

Add the banana mixture and refrigerate for 2 to 4 hours.

To serve, gently loosen the pudding from the sides of the dish by running a small knife around the inside of the ramekin.

Place a plate on top of the dish and invert.

(Note: It may be necessary to warm the bottom of the ramekin before inverting.)

Garnish with sliced bananas and a sprinkle of maple sugar and cinnamon.

Yield: 2 to 4 servings

GOLDEN STRAWBERRY BLUEBERRY CRUMBLE

½ cup spelt flour
½ cup rice flour
1 tablespoon arrowroot
1 cup date sugar, divided
2 tablespoons walnut oil
1 cup fresh or frozen blueberries
1 cup fresh or frozen strawberries
2 teaspoons freshly squeezed lemon juice
1 teaspoon ground cinnamon
1 tablespoon flaked coconut, fresh or packaged

Preheat the oven to 300° F.

In a large bowl, combine the flour, arrowroot, ½ cup date sugar, and walnut oil and blend using a fork or pastry blender.

Place blueberries and strawberries in a soufflé dish and mix in lemon juice, ½ cup date sugar, and cinnamon until berries are well-coated.

Cover berries evenly with the crumble mixture.

Place in the oven and bake for 15 to 20 minutes, or until golden brown.

Yield: 4 servings

CHILLED CANTALOUPE STUFFED WITH CHERRY CREAM
1 cup fresh or frozen cherries, pitted
½ teaspoon lemon extract
½ teaspoon almond extract
2 cups silken tofu
1 cantaloupe

Cut the cantaloupe in quarters. Remove the fruit from the peel, slice into bite-sized pieces, and return to the peel.

Combine the cherries, lemon extract, almond extract, and tofu in a food processor or blender and puree until smooth.

Place the cherry cream in a dessert dish and serve with the sliced cantaloupe.

Garnish with sliced lemon.

Yield: 4 servings

HOLIDAY GINGERBREAD
¾ cup oat flour
2 tablespoons arrowroot
1½ teaspoons baking powder
1 teaspoon ground cinnamon
1 teaspoon ground ginger
¼ teaspoon ground cloves
1 teaspoon ground nutmeg
½ cup apple butter
½ cup pure maple syrup

¼ cup almond milk
1 teaspoon orange extract
2 tablespoons walnut oil
½ cup walnuts

Preheat oven to 325° F.
In a large bowl, combine the flour, arrowroot, baking powder, cinnamon, ginger, cloves, and nutmeg.
In another bowl, combine the apple butter, maple syrup, almond milk, orange extract, and walnut oil and beat until smooth.
Fold the batter into the flour mixture, add the walnuts, and blend well.
Place in a greased loaf or baking pan and bake for 25 minutes or until a toothpick placed in the cake comes out clean.

OPTIONAL GLAZE:
2 cups confectioner's sugar
2 tablespoons almond milk
1 tablespoon maple syrup
½ teaspoon vanilla extract

Combine all ingredients in a bowl or blender and mix until smooth.

Drizzle glaze over top of the gingerbread.
Garnish with sliced figs, grated carrot, or walnuts.

Yield: 4 servings

Testimonials

The following testimonials are various first hand accounts by people who have successfully followed Gary's Null's natural protocols.

HOMEOPATHIC MEDICINE

Lillian on Rectal Cancer

Three years ago, I was diagnosed with a cancer below my rectum for which I received chemotherapy and radiation. That got rid of it for a while, but in time it reappeared in my liver. I received fifty chemotherapy treatments, but had I known what I understand today, I would never have had any.

I was very sick and waiting to die. I could not hold food or water down and lost a lot of weight. My bowels were totally paralyzed, and I could not go to the bathroom at all. The nurses told me I only had a short time to live, and I wanted to die. The pain was so bad that I had to live on morphine and a narcotic pain patch.

Thank God my daughter introduced me to a homeopathic doctor who gave me a new lease on life. My doctor has done an awful lot for me. My therapy consisted of a lot of natural herbs and vitamins. I juiced and ate a diet high in healthy vegetables. Red meats were eliminated. In addition, I received colonic therapy to detoxify my bowel.

When I got home, I had renewed strength. I could walk around and even drive, whereas before I needed a wheelchair. In six months, I have been able to gain some weight back and have no more bowel trouble. I had a myelogram last month. The doctors were shocked that I was able to come this far. They can't believe it. I am a totally different person. I am amazed and my whole family is amazed as well. I feel that if I didn't go there, I would be gone. If I had to do it over, I would not have chemotherapy or radiation at all. I would go the homeopathic route.

ESSIAC TEA

Marilyn on Breast Cancer

My husband brought home an article out of the newspaper about Essiac tea just before I had my lymph nodes removed. The doctors figured for sure that the lymph nodes were invaded with cancer. I started on this tea ten days before going back into the hospital. I went in and the lymph nodes and the rest of the surrounding tissues were clean. Three specialists were very surprised and kept remarking what a miracle it was because of the stage III cancer that had already broken free of the tumor and was already invading the rest of the breast.

Although I opted for a traditional approach to treatment, I attribute the lack of hair loss and the ability to handle radiation and chemotherapy without side effects to the benefits of the tea. I feel wonderful today. I've got a new lease on life. I drink the Essiac tea twice per day faithfully. This has been two years now.

Lynette on Bone Cancer

The prognosis was really bad. I went to see a bunch of specialists, and they basically all said the same thing: If I lived I wouldn't want to, because everything was just disintegrating. It was a big old mess, and I wasn't real happy because I wasn't able to get any answers.

I went to the health food store and started reading different books and talking to some people. That's how I learned about Essiac tea. I was kind of skeptical but got a number to find out what the deal was on this tea. I spoke to someone who told me that she had come across an all-natural herbal tea that doesn't affect any other medication that you're on. I said, "What the heck? I'll try it."

At the time, I could barely walk. I have total shoulder replacements and a hip replacement. The doctors tried doing bone grafts, but that didn't take. The disease was in my ankles, wrists, and knees. They wanted to do knee replacement surgery on me. In my situation, there is no stopping the disease, and there is no treatment for it. What they do is cut out the dead bone and try to put metal in there. I'm basically all bionic.

When I started drinking the tea, I could barely walk, I was on crutches, and my legs were swollen. I had them wrapped. I drank the tea three times per day. Within three to four days, I didn't have any pain.

I had some X-rays done before starting on the tea and afterward. Before the tea, they were really bad. My bones were fractured and broken, and all the ligaments were eaten away. Four weeks later, I had X-rays taken again. The doctor was amazed. The X-rays showed some bone damage, but not as much as before. A week later, I went to another doctor and had X-rays taken again. This was six weeks after taking the stuff. All the bone damage was gone. There was nothing there. They thought they mixed up my X-rays.

Today I'm great. I go biking and study martial arts. This stuff is great.

DR. NICHOLAS GONZALEZ'S ENZYME THERAPY

Edmund on Kidney Cancer

Four and a half years ago, I had major surgery. The doctors removed my left kidney, a large tumor, and one lymph node. I followed this with an interferon program for nine months to prevent any recurrence of the tumor. Unfortunately, this did not work for me, because a second tumor came back. At that time, the doctor said that even though kidney cancer does not respond to radiation or chemo, we should try radiation. The radiation stabilized the second tumor but did not make it disappear. At that time, I realized that the interferon was not going to work.

A friend of mine was on an aggressive nutritional program with Dr. Nicholas Gonzalez in New York City. I started this program three and a half years ago. Three months after I began the program, the second tumor disappeared. My weight, which was way down to 105, is now back to normal at 135. I'm feeling good. My color is back. And recent CT scans and bone scans have been negative. I'm seventy years old.

Henrietta on Breast Cancer with Metastases to the Lung

I had lymph node involvement and went through surgery. After six months of chemotherapy, I had a 50 percent chance of surviving five years. They never say anything about getting totally well, just five years. After three years, it metastasized around my left lung. At that point, the prognosis was not good. I was told that my life expectancy was two to three months.

At that point, I found Dr. Gonzalez in New York City. His treatment is a three-part program consisting of supplements, diet and detoxification. I have been going to Dr. Gonzalez for three years and nine months.

The program has been very successful for me. I can't say it is an easy program. It requires a lot of self-discipline because the diet is rigorous. I'm not saying that you just start on this program and feel great. You don't. If anything, I felt worse before I felt better, because of the toxicity that was built up in my body. But it has worked for me, and I believe so strongly in the program that it has taken the fear of cancer away. I think this may be a major key to my recovery, because when you believe in something that strongly, it takes fear away.

At this point, I am stabilized. My cancer level is down to a safe zone, and I am functioning normally. I feel great. My oncologist said that if indeed I was still alive, I was a very lucky woman. They didn't give me any hope of living with the traditional medicine.

GERSON THERAPY

Tom on Skin Melanoma

In March 1982, I found a mole on the right side of my forehead. It didn't concern me much because it wasn't big; it was about half the size of my little fingernail. I talked to my family physician about it, not thinking much of it, but when he saw the thing, he was concerned. He said, "We'd better take this off and biopsy it."

They did that, and the report that came back really shocked me, because I had been eating organic foods and a right diet for many years. The news was all bad. It was malignant, it was Clark Level 4. . . .

After the surgery, the cancer returned within ten days to the site of the incision. I guess that was because they didn't get it all. Then I began to have tumors appearing all over my upper body, chest, and arm. This all happened within a matter of days.

Initially, they wanted to do extensive surgery at the site of the original appearance, but when the thing spread, four different doctors started giving me different advice. Basically, they were all saying that nothing was going to cure this cancer.

At that point, I declined the radical surgery that they wanted to do on the site of my head, and I started looking for different approaches. I knew something about alternative methods, but nobody was at all hopeful, until we talked to the Gerson people. We called the Gerson Institute, and they said that the Gerson therapy was very effective against melanomas. They said that the fact that I hadn't had other treatments that would tend to suppress the immune system was in my favor. I knew something about the therapy, so it wasn't a complete shock. I had some belief in Dr. Gerson and his therapy, so I tried it.

I talked to Charlotte [Gerson Straus], and she said that melanoma patients detoxify rapidly. She said my chances of recovery were good, but that I would have quite a bit of nausea in the beginning. Everything she told me came true. I got quite ill initially, the type of illness that you'd have if you had a stomach flu. But I was nervous enough about my situation that after I had been on the therapy for a week or so, I thought, my God, I'm not going to be able to do this.

The family had a council of war. We all talked it over with the Institute. They calmed me down and told me they'd cut back the juices a little bit, and cut back the medicine a little for a few days, and just keep trying it. We got through that period, and I felt better again.

The heart and soul of the Gerson therapy is that every hour of the day, from eight o'clock in the morning to seven at night, you have an 8-ounce glass of fresh-squeezed vegetable and fruit juice. It alternates. Basically, one hour you have a juice that's half carrot juice mixed with apple juice, and the next hour you have green juice, which I think is three different types of lettuce, plus green pepper, red cabbage, and then apple with that also. The juices are laced with potassium salts. In addition, you have three meals. The Gerson therapy is not a fast at all, but your diet is specified.

In the beginning of the therapy, you start digesting the cancer and putting it out of the body in the form of metabolic toxins. If your body is full of cancer the way mine was, you're going to have a lot of toxins to process. To help that out, in the beginning. . . you take a coffee enema every four hours when you're up: 6:00 a.m., 10:00 a.m., 2:00 p.m., 6:00 p.m., and 10:00 p.m. The coffee enemas put the drug caffeine directly into the portal vein. That enables the liver to detoxify a lot more efficiently than it could otherwise. The coffee enema is a great help. It relieves pain, it relieves digestive discomfort, and it is a crucial part of the therapy. That's basically how it went in a day.

Within two months, every visible tumor on my body had regressed. They had shrunk, dried up, and fallen off. It all happened so quickly. I started out in March 1982 thinking I was a healthy guy. Then, in early May 1982, I was told that I had cancer and very little chance to live. In July 1982, I was on the Gerson therapy, and everything cancerous that could be seen had regressed and disappeared. The Gerson people said that even though everything that could be seen was gone, there was more of a problem under the surface. They recommended that I stay on the therapy for eighteen to twenty-four months, which I did. I stayed on the therapy for twenty months, and in the subsequent thirteen years, I've had no recurrence of the cancer.

Over the years, I've talked to hundreds of people with cancer of various types, and I try to share my experience with them. You can pretty much see who will succeed with this type of therapy and who will not. People used to the passive mode, where professionals do things to them—they cut, they burn, and they put chemicals in, and the patients sit there while it happens to them—are generally horrified when they find out the extent to which the patient has to cooperate in his own recovery on one of these metabolic programs. But people who can take that aboard have a very, very high success rate on this therapy. The exceptions are people who have been bombed with chemotherapy before they get on it. In order to do the Gerson therapy, you have to be motivated and open to radical change in lifestyle that a diet change like this imposes.

Joan on Breast Cancer

I had a radical mastectomy. One year later, I had a recurrence. I was not biopsied, however. The surgeon said that he would monitor this mass.

My husband and I did a lot of research and decided to try the Gerson therapy. I began the program in August 1977. By May 1978, when I saw the surgeon again, the mass was gone. Since that time, I have remained completely clear. It has been eighteen years, and I have never had any recurrences. I have had myself closely monitored over the years by surgeons and lab work.

The Gerson therapy is intensive and comprehensive. It consists of nutritional treatment through diet and thirteen juices per day. It consists of medication, potassium, niacin, thyroid, lugol solution, pancreatin, acidol pepsin, and liver and B12 combined as daily injections. It also consists of detoxification in the form of coffee enemas to help the liver. It's a very comprehensive therapy.

I still continue with my diet of organically grown fruits and vegetables. I also continue with almost daily coffee enemas. I have not eaten meat, except for poultry and fish, for these eighteen years. That was a decision I made on my own. Some people go back to their former diets, but I realized that my former diet was too high in fats and could be a possible problem again.

I did not tell the surgeon that I was doing the Gerson therapy. Nor did he ask me any questions. I wanted to keep the surgeon monitoring me, so I decided not to make him angry by telling him what I had done.

At the time, there was not the knowledge and the education about any options as far as treatment was concerned, except for the orthodox establishment options. I had been told at the beginning about the American Cancer Society's statistics and what their thoughts on treatment were. I was an R.N. who saw that much of this treatment was ineffective with the cancer patients, so I did not feel that the American Cancer Society was credible. Having seen this in my profession, I decided that I was going to do a different therapy. I had read about Gerson's therapy in Dr. Gerson's book. I felt it was credible and the thing to do for myself.

Patricia on Pancreatic Cancer

I had pancreatic cancer that spread to my liver, gallbladder, and spleen, and was told that I had less than three months to live. My doctors were doing nothing. They said that chemotherapy and anything else would not help me and that I should prepare my family and get my affairs in order. I was in the process of doing that. Then, one morning, my husband and I heard about the Gerson clinic in

Mexico. My husband got up and said, "That's it. Pack your clothes. We're going."

We went down on March 7, 1986, and started the therapy that day. Before I started the therapy, I had been throwing up mouthfuls of blood. I was just about finished. Ten days later, I stopped bringing up blood, and the pain was gone. I said to my husband, "I don't know if I'm going to live, but I feel better than I have in a year."

Six months later, I went to see my doctor, who wondered why I was still around. He asked if I would have a CT scan, which I did. The test showed that the masses of cancer had gone. My doctor said, "I don't know what you're doing, and I don't want to know what you're doing, but just keep doing it." I think he was shocked to see that I was still around.

Another six months down the road, he asked me to take another CT scan, which I did. He said, "Patricia, there's no sign of cancer at all." That was nine years ago. Today, I feel wonderful. I have no sign of cancer at all.

I took the two Gerson books to my doctor, and he read them, but he said that it was just too deep for him. He just calls me his miracle now.

Marilyn on Melanoma and Cervical Cancer

I developed these conditions in 1979 when I was thirty-six years of age. My prognosis from my physicians was not good. The melanoma, in particular, was very virulent. They didn't come out and tell me how long they thought I had to live, but they tactfully tried to tell me that my chances weren't good. I read and did some of my own research and found that with stage IV melanoma, the patient tends to expire in one to five years. It's now been fifteen years. I'm not a typical patient.

I did a lot of research and picked Dr. Max Gerson's therapy because I felt that it was the hardest and the most curative. It had the best results with melanoma. I was inspired by the fact that Dr. Gerson had worked with Albert Schweitzer, and that he was a pioneer. He just was an incredible physician with a wonderful answer, but not many people were willing to use his therapy for their problems.

I found that after the first six months of the therapy, I began to feel really normal. I didn't have reactions and feelings that come when you do a metabolic therapy. I started to feel intuitively that I wasn't going to die—that I was never going to have a recurrence. I know that the mind has a great deal to do with healing. I just knew because this diet was building my cells that my mind was stronger. I felt that I had turned the corner. It's been almost sixteen years, and I feel better than I ever have in my life. I attribute that to Dr. Gerson's work and, of course, my participating in it.

Sharon on Non-Hodgkin's Lymphoma

I did not have chemotherapy. I went directly to the Gerson Hospital. I was there for two weeks, and in five days I lost twenty-eight pounds of fluid. I had been very swollen with edema. When I got back, I continued on the therapy, and in six months I went back to the doctor. I had an MRI, and my tumor was gone. I am not on a modified therapy. It's been three years.

George on Pancreatic Cancer

I went to the Gerson therapy center in February 1983. Prior to going there, my wife and I were on the way to Hawaii. We were in Seattle and preparing to leave for Hawaii the next morning. I got very sick and had a lot of pain in my stomach and back. We phoned the doctor who was listed in the hotel directory, and took a taxi to the hospital. I had a blood test, an X-ray, and an examination by a doctor there. The doctor said that he wasn't sure what the problem was, but he suggested that we not go to Hawaii. He said we should go home instead and get further tests done. That's what we did.

My doctor sent me to a specialist in Victoria. I went through a lot of tests that I had never heard of before. On January 21, the specialist took some blood tests and said that the amylase in my blood was high. A normal level was between 70 and 320, and mine was 627. It proved that there was a very bad infection in my body.

I finally took a CT scan, which showed a mass in the head of the pancreas. The specialist said that there was absolutely no question about it. I had cancer of the pancreas.

We had heard about Gerson's therapy through somebody my daughter knew. We phoned the Gerson Institute and went down there in February 1983. We spent one month there.

Afterward, we stayed in our condo in Escondido for eight months, because that was the only place we could get organic foods. We had our organic vegetables delivered by a lady who got her vegetables from the same source as the Gersons.

When we came home, I had put weight on, and I felt good. My blood tests were also good. I took another CT scan, and it showed no tumor. I phoned the head doctor at Gerson's in April 1984, and he told me to stay another four months on the program . . . . That was eleven years ago, and I have had absolutely no problem since.

REVICI THERAPY

Fernando on Prostate Cancer

I was diagnosed for prostate cancer at age fifty-six. I scored 8 on the Gleason scale, which I understand is rather high. The cells were highly undifferentiated, which I understand makes them proliferate more rapidly. And I was also at a relatively young age to get prostate cancer. Those three things, everyone seemed to agree, would make it more aggressive. My urologist immediately suggested a radical prostatectomy. I declined, for two reasons, because I was not and am not convinced that invasive therapies lengthen the lifespan, and on the other hand, they do alter your lifestyle tremendously, and I was not ready to undergo the changes that operations of that sort apparently cause you. After some research, I decided to come to Dr. Revici, and I'm very happy that I did.

I've also made changes to my lifestyle, nutritionally and with supplementation. I've started to take ozone therapy. Basically, what Dr. Revici's therapy did to an extremely aggressive carcinoma is apparently to have stopped it in its tracks. From what I've heard from mainstream doctors and urologists tell me, the way it seemed from the outset was that I did not have much time—two and a half or three years. Here I am, with lots of energy and very enthusiastic to the response my body has had to Dr. Revici's therapy. I've been in remission five years, and I hope we can extend that indefinitely.

Joseph on Pancreatic Cancer

I had cancer of the pancreas. My prognosis was not good. The surgeon told me to go to the Lord and pray for a miracle, and that was it. I had three to six months to live, and I tried the chemotherapy. And then I was put in touch with Dr. Revici, and once that happened, I stopped chemotherapy. I stayed on his therapy until now—that was ten years ago. I do not have pancreatic cancer now. I've been cured.

Charlotte on Ovarian and Oat Cell Lung Cancer

In 1980, I was diagnosed with ovarian cancer and oat cell lung cancer. I had a hysterectomy and started on chemotherapy. I really was not pleased with chemotherapy and was looking around for something else. When I came to Dr. Revici, I went off chemotherapy and started taking a sulfur drug he had in capsules. I took that drug for about six months. When I went off chemotherapy, I was told the cancer would return by the end of the month and that I would be dead in six months. After six months, I had an X-ray done, and there was no sign of any lung tumor, and I've never had any reoccurrence. Now sixteen years later, I'm still cancer-free through Dr. Revici's treatments.

Norman on Colon Cncer

Over six years ago, I had surgery for colon cancer. The doctors didn't have any recommendations; they said I was on my own.

I heard about Dr. Revici and decided to see him. It's probably the best thing I have done in many, many years. I went on his program, which consists mostly of minerals. At first it was rather intense in that I had to use them four times per day, but like everything else, you get used to it.

Now I'm on a maintenance program where I use his prescribed minerals one month on and six months off. My CEA test, which is the test that they use for colon cancer, comes in below 0.5. I only need to have a colonoscopy every two years because I've been clear for several years. I'm just happy to be here. I only have praise for him.

Robert on Angiosarcoma

I discovered that I had a lump in my jaw. I went through a series of extensive tests, including two biopsies, one in the hospital and one outside. It included MRIs, CT scans, X-rays, and that sort of thing. Out of that came the diagnosis of angiosarcoma. Basically, the doctor who was associated with Georgetown Hospital told me that with this diagnosis I had about one chance in ten of being alive in five years. He said that that particular kind of cancer was not treatable by any of the usual techniques, namely surgery, radiation, or chemotherapy.

Given that kind of prognosis, and given the lack of treatment options, I decided it was time to look elsewhere for treatment. My wife had worked with a lady who was a former patient of Dr. Revici, so I knew of Dr. Revici through her and contacted the doctor. I was actively under his care for about six years. By that I mean I went to see him in his office approximately once a month. The treatment consisted primarily of capsules that I took orally. He put me on a number of different medications.

What struck me about his treatment is that he tailors it to the person. He would sometimes have me on two or three medications. He would tell me to call him in three or four days, and he might change the medication, depending upon how I was reacting to it. Over that period, he probably had me on a couple dozen different things. I have not been receiving treatment for a little over a year.

His office asked me to have an MRI done, which I did, and a couple of months ago, I sent them the results. Basically, the MRI shows that in the last three years, there has been no growth at all in the tumor.

Jay on Squamous Cell Carcinoma

I had a squamous cell carcinoma in the throat and was given two to six months to live. They wanted to operate and remove my entire voice box—my vocal cords and everything—and give me chemo, which I wouldn't allow.

I immediately got on Dr. Revici's therapy and studied his entire program relating not only to his medication, but also to the nutrition, vitamins, minerals, enzymes, and even some bioactive frequencies later on.

That was thirteen years ago. Today, I feel like a million dollars. I have never spent a night in the hospital. I'm very active. At the time I started on his program, you couldn't understand me. I sounded like the Godfather's godfather. In a period of about four months, my voice was back to normal, and I've never had a sick day.

I've spoken with my original diagnosing physicians many, many times. I happened to know one in New York, and one in California, who are top guys in the allopathic field in otolaryngology. About two years later, I finally agreed to let them do a second in-depth biopsy on my throat, just to get them off my back, because they were friends of mine. When my right vocal cord was originally diagnosed, it was over three-quarters of an inch in diameter. They couldn't understand why all of this cleared up in such a short period of time. It was all 100 percent clear.

Arthur on Kaposi's Sarcoma

I was diagnosed at the VA hospital. The doctors there suggested operating to cut out the sores on my foot. I did not agree. I didn't like the approach they had there.

I decided I would try another method. Fortunately, I listened to you and learned about Dr. Revici. I began treatment with him back in 1991. I successfully overcame my condition.

Lee on Breast Cancer

My cancer started in 1986. I felt a lump in the right breast, and had a mammogram, which was negative. The doctor said that the lump was benign, and that I shouldn't worry. In 1988, the lump seemed bigger and harder, and I was advised again to get a mammogram. This time, it showed a mass. I then had a biopsy at Beth Israel Hospital, which diagnosed a 4 cm infiltrating ductal carcinoma in my breast. I saw a number of doctors and surgeons who advised a modified radical mastectomy, with chemotherapy and radiation.

I knew that there were other options from listening to your program and reading. I decided to try Dr. Revici's nontoxic individualized cancer therapy, even though I was warned by all the doctors that he was a quack, and that I could die without conventional treatment. I had the lumpectomy in December 1988, and I began treatment with Dr. Revici in January 1989.

I found him to be very caring and considerate. He encouraged me to call him often to tell him how I was feeling. His own phone number was given to me.

In July 1989, I stopped the treatment because I felt that six months of it was sufficient. About nine months later, I felt another lump in the same breast. A mammogram revealed another mass, approximately 1.5 cm, and the tumor marker for breast cancer was high.

I returned to Dr. Revici in May 1990, and he urged me to have the lump removed. I didn't want another operation, and Dr. Revici was understanding. He said that he would try to help me anyway.

I was given a variety of Dr. Revici's medicine. At times I became discouraged, but Dr. Revici kept reassuring me that the lump would go away. Gradually, it did become softer, and after about two years, I no longer felt the lump.

The last mammogram I had was negative, and the tumor marker for breast cancer was normal. I still take Dr. Revici's medicine about every two months. I also take vitamins and herbs. I changed my diet. I don't have meat or chicken, and I eat very little sugar or dairy. I drink bottled water and take exercise classes in yoga and low-impact aerobics. I am very grateful to Dr. Revici.

Ronald on Bone, Lung, and Kidney Cancer

My experience with cancer began in 1976, when a large tumor was discovered in my pelvis just above the knee. It resulted in an amputation in 1977. In 1979, the cancer metastasized to the lung, and I had an operation on my right lung to remove a couple of nodules. To my regret, in 1980, I was diagnosed with renal cell carcinoma. At that time, they told me that I had six months to two years to live. There was no treatment available. Surgery wasn't possible. Neither was chemotherapy expected to be of any benefit.

At that point, I heard about Dr. Revici, and went to see him. I started on his therapy in October 1980. To my surprise, within about a month or so, I began to feel my energy return. My appetite began to increase, and my condition improved. I continued on his therapy for a while. Then I returned to work.

I had another episode of metastatic cancer in 1987. Again the bone cancer was active in my left hip. I went back to Dr. Revici. With his help, I went into remission. Unfortunately, in 1991, I had another episode of bone and lung cancer. I went back to Dr. Revici again, and have continued on his therapy until today. The tumor in the right lung was a little resistant to the treatment, but after a couple of years of treatment, it appears that the tumor is going into remission. I'm very happy about that.

I've been able to enjoy a reasonable quality of life over these years, thanks to Dr. Revici's treatment. My life certainly has been extended beyond the six months to two years that was expected by the traditional medical community.

DR. STANISLAW BURZYNSKI'S ANTINEOPLASTON THERAPY

Theresa on Stage IV Lymphoma

In 1984, after the birth of my daughter, I had a biopsy that showed that I had stage IV lymphoma. My doctors said that I should go on chemotherapy right away, even though I wouldn't be able to get rid of the lymphoma. They said it was incurable.

I had a second opinion . . . and they said the same thing, but they said they could check it for a while and not give me any chemo right away. I never did end up having chemotherapy or radiation.

Today, I'm great, thanks to Dr. Burzynski. He gave me the antineoplaston therapy, which means anticancer. It's a peptide that he discovered. Apparently, most peptides are growth-enhancing peptides. Peptides are precursors to amino acids, which are the precursors to proteins. The peptides that he found are peptides that inhibit the growth of certain types of cells. Rather than killing the cancer cells along with a lot of other healthy cells, peptides just keep the cancer cells from growing. They live out their lifespan, and then they die off. Eventually, whatever organ is affected is turned back into a healthy organ. That's what happened with me.

While I was healing, I made a lot of changes. I realized I had a lot of anger that I wasn't dealing with. I was taught that anger is bad and hurtful, and I developed a way of suppressing my anger while not even knowing that I had it. So one part of getting well, a big part, was coming more to terms with my anger, accepting it, and expressing it appropriately, rather than stuffing it inside and turning it into cancer.

Another aspect was learning to visualize my cancer going away, and holding a more positive view of my future. I did change a lot of things. I changed my job, and I changed a lot of my relationships. I went through a lot of changes.

Today, I feel a lot different than I did then. I'm much more aware of my feelings, and physically I feel a lot better. Over the months that

I worked with Dr. Burzynski's medicine, I saw my cancer gradually disappear. I was grateful to be able to deal with my healing process in a nontoxic way, and I'm really grateful to be alive.

Venuta on Breast Cancer

One week after diagnosis, I had a mastectomy. Then they wanted to give me chemotherapy, but I didn't want it. I decided to go to Dr. Burzynski. He connected me to an IV for five months, non-stop, twenty-four hours per day with his anti-neoplaston medication. During that time, I was never sick. I had a normal life. I have a seven-year-old child. I've been going to meetings at school. I've been driving my car. I have chemotherapy, and I can drive my car. I never even lost my hair. Nobody in the whole world knew that I was having chemotherapy. After five years. I am talking with you.

Currently, I am perfect. I have no cancer. I feel good, and I run my own business. I go to Dr. Burzynski for check-ups, and everything looks good.

Ellen on Intestinal Asbestos Cancer

This is the same type of cancer that Steve McQueen died of. It was a slow-growing cancer. I was on 250 pain pills a month for ten years. Finally, Sloan-Kettering gave me two years to live. I called Dr. Burzynski and asked him if he could help me. After the first week of treatment, I was off the pain pills. I had no side effects. I was on his program for nine months, and I got cured.

Tessie on Lymphoma

I was advised to get chemotherapy, which I started in June 1992. In July 1993, it reappeared in my neck. My doctor said that with my condition, chemotherapy might help. But the second time that I started chemotherapy, the tumor was not getting smaller.

I had the feeling that I had to do something different. I decided to go to Dr. Burzynski because I got tired of the chemotherapy. I told my doctor that I was going to stop the chemotherapy and get a second opinion. My doctor was shocked, and he started putting pressure on me to go back on chemotherapy. He said I would lose ground, but I didn't. Today, I am free of cancer.

Actually, the chemotherapy was causing me to lose ground. I was so weak from it that I was running a fever. I had bronchitis, and I had pneumonia. My heart was also damaged from the chemotherapy. After getting well, I went back to my doctor for blood tests to send to Dr. Burzynski, and he was ignoring me.

Mary Jo on Low-Grade Non-Hodgkin's Lymphoma, Stage IV

I was told that I needed a bone marrow transplant, massive chemotherapy, total body irradiation, and six weeks of total isolation in a hospital. My doctor gave me no guarantee, but he said that this was my only chance for a cure. My other option was to take chemotherapy and radiation every two years. I already had a tumor on the side of my neck, which was growing. If I didn't follow his advice, he said it would press against my organs and I would die.

I did some more research. That's when I heard about Dr. Burzynski's totally nontoxic treatment. I thought I would be foolish not to try it. When I called my doctor at UCLA, he was adamant that I not start Dr. Burzynski's treatment, but I did it anyway.

My medical records are open to everybody. Every CT scan I had showed a reduction. I have maintained my doctor at UCLA who says, over and over again, "I can't say it's not working, but I don't know why it's working." He calls me a spontaneous remission.

One thing that is so important about Dr. Burzynski's treatment is that it is totally nontoxic. I lived a completely normal life while I was on it. I was able to do grocery shopping, drive my kid's car pools, everything.

DR. GARY NULL'S PROTOCOLS

Murray

I have always respected Gary's work and looked forward to a worth-while experience. I am a psychotherapist and had reservations about Chi Gong, but I thought that it had merit. Breathwork and Physique were marvelous, as was learning power walking up hills. Since the retreat, I continue to meditate and use technique exercises. I had previously been diagnosed with bladder cancer, and making these changes has caused it to reverse.

I am grateful for the retreat experience, lectures, and support groups, and I plan on passing on the information I learned from the lectures to my patients.

Nina

I was diagnosed with lung cancer. I was anemic and had arthritis, almost no energy, and elevated blood pressure. Pain went through me when I walked. I underwent radiation, chemotherapy, and body scans.

I was ready for a life change but was not certain where to go or whom to see. After hearing Gary Null on television and radio, I was curious and joined a health support group. I ate flesh foods and used dairy.

Today I am vegan. I drink green juices and follow the protocol completely. I am cancer-free without medication. My arthritis has diminished, and I can use and enjoy my body by walking, doing yoga, and working in the wardrobe department of a theatrical company. I look forward to a good season with the crew. I am delighted with the results of each new blood test. I have developed personal insight.

Adele

I was a cancer patient. I had frequent illnesses. I had no energy. I was very tired. Entering a support group gave me hope, and I followed the protocol. I enjoyed it and my group companions. Today, the cancer is in remission. The protocol helped detox this condition. I maintain a more positive attitude and completed a New York marathon. I do not get sick frequently anymore and find I have much more energy.

Alim

Three of the tumors I once had are no more; another one has decreased in size. My skin is softer and smoother. My stomach is smaller. I feel more energetic. I exercise regularly.

Grace

The biggest change that has impacted me is that my breast cancer is now gone. There are no indications of any cancer. My vision has also improved since I started using Gary Null's Anti-Aging Vitamins.

Etta

Before—She had a hysterectomy for uterine cancer, but the cancer returned. She went through chemotherapy and radiation. She had arthritis, psoriasis, and low energy, and she was overweight and unhappy at work.

After—Her cancer seems to be in full remission. She lost twenty-six pounds. Her psoriasis is gone. Her hair and skin are healthy, her arthritis is gone, and her immune system is strong.

It was through class assignments and other workbook activities that she learned she was hard on herself and came to experience the positive relief of forgiveness of self and others.

Etta left her toxic job. She meditates twice daily, exercises, practices yoga, and lifts weights.

DR. LAWRENCE BURTON'S THERAPY

Craig on Lymphoma

I was originally diagnosed in 1979 with a malignant lymphoma. By the time it was diagnosed, it was already stage IV, which meant that it was in my bones.

I was given radiation and three different series of chemotherapy in early 1980. When they saw how my liver was, they gave me a 10 percent chance of seeing Christmas Day. I continued on more radiation and chemotherapy.

In the meantime, I saw a program on *60 Minutes* about Dr. Lawrence Burton in the Bahamas and how he was blackballed from the medical establishment. He was being recognized as a viable cancer researcher. I kept it in the back of my mind.

I kept getting worse and worse and worse. Finally, I went to the Bahamas as a last resort. The treatment I received was a daily injection of four different proteins. There were absolutely no side effects whatsoever. I began to feel better right away. Of course, I'd been through a lot of chemotherapy, and I was coming out of that. It took me about a year to really start coming back, but everything has been fine. I've had a lot of check-ups ever since, and there's absolutely no sign of cancer in my body.

Jesse on Lymphoma

In 1980, I was diagnosed with lymphoma. I had twenty treatments of radiation, and eleven months of chemotherapy. During this time, the cancer continued to spread. It spread to both lungs, and to the bone marrow. During this two years of treatment, I had many biopsies done, which all turned out to be malignant tumors. After the two years, they told me to come back in two weeks, and they would tell me what they were going to do next, but that I had very little time left, and they were going to try to make me as comfortable as they could.

When I came home, I knew I was not going back, because I had heard of this place in Freeport, Bahamas. I called a lady, and she gave me a phone number to reach the Bahamas. I called, and they took me. I had to bring my records, which the doctors did not want me to have, but they couldn't hold me, so they gave me very little information to take with me.

I went to Freeport in June 1982. When I went, I really didn't go for a cure, because I had been told that I had a very short time left. I could look at myself and I knew that, because I had tumors all over my body and on my face. I was covered from top to bottom.

After going to Freeport, Dr. Burton told me that the lymphoma that I had, chemo would not even treat. After he told me that, I knew that he was telling the truth because it had continued to spread.

After being in Freeport for just a few days, I had a talk with Dr. Burton, and after talking with him, I knew that he had the cure. He said to me, "You don't have a problem." That in itself did so much for me, because you will have a tendency to believe what a doctor tells you. There I sat, barely able to hold my head up, and Dr. Burton was telling me that I didn't have a problem.

After two weeks, all of the visible tumors were gone. After one week, I could see a great difference in the way that I felt. And after five weeks, I was sent home. It was in July 1982.

When I came back, I saw my treating physician. He said that I was cured, but that it was the chemo that cured me. He twisted his story because I had five biopsies just before leaving his care and going to the Bahamas, and they were all malignant. He did the biopsies, and he gave me the reports, telling me that he was going to make me as comfortable as he could before I died. Yet, when I came home from Freeport, he told me that I was cured.

That, in itself, makes me very bitter, knowing that a doctor will lie to you, and tell you just anything. I really don't appreciate that. To me, cancer in the United States is just a money racket. I know what they took from me, and they gave me nothing. I would love to have a refund.

714-X THERAPY

Susan on Her Son's Hodgkin's Disease

Last summer, Billy was diagnosed with Hodgkin's disease. We didn't know any better, so we went with chemotherapy. Billy had five treatments from August until October. Although he did fairly well compared to some people, he did have the typical side effects. He got nauseous and tired, he lost his hair, and he had some jaw pain. His main concern with the chemotherapy was that it was poisonous. He would look at the drugs dripping into his body and realize how toxic they were. That, in a nutshell, is why he ran away.

When we started to talk about using other forms of treatment, the doctors began to use scare tactics on us. They told us that Billy would die if he went off chemotherapy, and they described to Billy, in detail, exactly how he would die. They said that in addition to the chemotherapy, Billy would have to have radiation at the end of the treatment program. Billy refused any more treatment.

We were contacted by many people about many therapies. One of these people, Charles Pixley of Writers and Research in Rochester, New York, told us about a therapy called 714-X. Initially, he sent us a booklet about the treatment. Eventually, Billy, my husband and I decided to use it. That was in January, and Billy has since flourished. His cancer is gone. Last December, he was tested, and there was some cancer at that point. In March, he was tested again, and the cancer was totally gone. He continues with the treatment. They recommend a six-month minimum treatment. We're almost at the end of that.

Billy is flourishing with this therapy. His hair has come back. He has gained weight. He has grown. He is like a vacuum cleaner as far as his appetite goes. He is a very active young man. He loves skateboarding, and skateboards every day if weather permits.

The doctors who originally said he would have been dead more or less pat us on the back and say that's nice. Instead of expressing interest, they tried to force us into continuing with chemotherapy by reporting us to the Department of Social Services. However, no action was ever taken, and we were able to pursue the treatment of our choice.

I have informed the media about our story in an attempt to get on national TV. I want to tell them about 714-X and where to get it, because we get hundreds of calls from people all over who have searched for it.

The media is apparently afraid, because they all appear interested when I call them, but I never hear back from them.

Harry on Massive Tumor outside Colon

I was given six months to a year to live. The surgeon said for me to live it up, and eat and do anything I wanted to do. He sent me to the oncologist, who told me that they could give me treatments but that I had about a 15 percent chance of being helped, and even if I was helped, the treatments would only increase my longevity by a couple of months. I was discouraged with that, so I made some trips to Mexico to study various alternative treatment approaches. Then I got a newsletter from a friend of mine about 714-X and I decided to try it because it was something I felt I could continue on.

My son gave me the injections, which were painless. We followed this program for six months. The total program consisted of 168 shots. Right after I started taking the 714-X, I felt better. I feel just fine now.

When I started on this program, my son turned my way of living around 180 degrees. He prepared an organic diet for me. I cut out alcohol and cut down on cigar smoking to one in the morning and one at night.

Since then, I have felt much better than I have in years. The 714-X stimulated my immune system back to normal.

I went back to my doctor two years later and was given a colonoscopy and some other tests. Tests showed that the tumor had not enlarged and that the growth had stopped. It became dormant. The oncologist wanted to see me, I guess, out of curiosity. He told me that I have a 60 percent better chance of survival. He said that, eventually, the tumor will shrink and then disappear.

Rick on Leukemia

At first, I tried chemotherapy, but it failed to work five times. After each treatment, I would experience a relapse because my leukemia was so aggressive. I was working on my next option, a bone marrow transplant. Iowa City had a few matches for me. The first one they tested was almost a perfect match, so I went in and had the transplant done. They gave me a 5 percent chance of actually making it through the transplant. Even if I made it through the transplant, I only had another 5 percent chance of cure. I survived the transplant but, three months later; my blood tests were really bad. My platelets never did recover completely.

I continued looking for answers. I was very familiar with Reich's technology and felt strongly that something along those lines could help me. The only problem was that nobody was using or dealing with this technology.

I had a live cell blood analysis done, which tells you more than a CBC or any test given in conventional medicine. According to my test, it was obvious that I was relapsing from the transplant. My relapse wasn't documented by conventional medicine, but, of course, they don't use this method, so it doesn't matter. I knew, and other people knew.

Eventually, I found a group that was duplicating what Reich did with his ray tube. I found this machine, got the 714-X again, and went back on these alternative therapies. Three weeks after getting this machine and getting back on the 714-X, my blood counts, every single one of them, returned to within the normal range. It was amazing. Everybody was astounded by it. I don't know what to attribute it to, but I do know that something helped me. I had my transplant in January 1994. I recovered around April, and here it is May 1995. I've had normal blood tests ever since.

COMBINATION THERAPIES AND LIFESTYLE CHANGES

Ed on Prostate Cancer

I had a radical prostatectomy. Afterward, my PSA kept going up. It got to 9.1. They thought it would be in the lymph nodes, and they wanted to do chemo and radiation. At that point, I was pretty disgusted; I wanted to try some alternative approaches. I went for hypnotherapy. I also started working with a dietitian to change my diet. I started eating whole foods: fruits, vegetables, foods that weren't processed. I ate more organic foods.

This was a big change for me, because I was brought up on meat and potatoes. It was also difficult for me because I grew up not liking vegetables. As a child, my mother forced us to eat what was on our plates, which included spinach and Brussels sprouts and broccoli, and I didn't even like being in the same room as a Brussels sprout. So I had a lot of changing to do.

I also started Essiac tea. When I started on the tea and the diet, it started moving my PSA down. It's down to 0.1 now, the normal range. I feel as healthy as a horse.

Cathy on Stage IV Hodgkin's Disease

I was in such bad shape that I couldn't lay down or walk. There was fluid in my lungs and tumors around my heart, which advanced into my abdomen. I had been on chemotherapy for about ten months. At first, the chemo got me back on my feet, but after a while it stopped working. That's when the doctors recommended a bone marrow transplant. They said it was my only hope for long-term survival.

At that point, I simply could not tolerate any more chemotherapy, and the thought of a bone marrow transplant was out of the question. I had heard about 714-X from a very well-respected physician in British Colombia, and I decided to start it. At the same time, I began to follow a holistic program.

I made quite a few changes. I had always thought that I had a healthy lifestyle, but I learned that, in fact, it really wasn't. I started doing everything that I could do to strengthen my immune system. That included a completely chemical-free lifestyle and an organic diet, with no white sugar or flour and very little dairy. The little dairy that I did have was unpasteurized and organic. I also had a lot of fresh vegetable juice and used only distilled water. I was also very careful about using chemical-free skin and hair products and about avoiding toxins such as household cleaners and pesticides. Along with that, I was on a very strict detoxification program which included cell cleanses, gallbladder flushes, and coffee enemas. I exercised using a trampoline and took pancreatic enzymes and glandulars that were specifically prescribed for me by a holistic physician. Altogether, it did the trick, and now I'm completely clear.

I began to notice improvement two to three weeks into the program. My energy level increased, and I had less pain. The best way to describe it is to say that I started to feel like my old self again. Two months after starting the 714-X, I had a CT scan done, and it showed marked improvement, so I knew I was on the right track. I was very excited. On my latest scan, which I just had last month, it showed that there was no sign of disease at all. I feel wonderful.

The most important thing is to have hope no matter what your physician tells you. You have to believe that there is more out there. You can fight for your life. I did, and it worked. It's just a matter of getting the right information. I think it's important to get information from both the medical side as well as the holistic side and find out what is best for you and what you believe in. Then go for it. Put everything into it that you can, and it will work.

Karina on Breast Cancer

I was diagnosed with breast cancer two years ago, and they gave me six months to live. I did the chemotherapy. I did four surgeries, and nothing worked. I felt like I was going to die. I decided to do something different and run away from the doctors. I did macrobiotics for two years. I changed my life completely. I changed my diet. I used to eat bad food—ice cream and meat—now I eat vegetables, at least five green per a day, and all kinds of supplements. I eat beans, tofu, and tempeh, and drink vitamin C. I dance eight hours per day and have a lot of energy. I still have the tumor, but it's going away.

Orville on Lymphoma that Had Metastasized

I am sixty-six years old and had always enjoyed good health until two years ago, when a bump appeared over my right temple. It started growing fast and was about the size of a marble. It was removed, and I was told that I had an aggressive non-Hodgkin's small cell lymphoma. I was interested in alternative medicine, and that's the route I took. First I went to Mexico for treatment, and it disappeared in about three weeks. I thought that was fantastic since I had arrived with cancer all over my body.

A few months later it began to appear again. I went to Dr. Michael Schachter's clinic in Suffern, New York. After a couple of weeks of treatments there, it vanished again.

Then it came back a third time, months later. At one point, the cancer got as large as a golf ball on my jawbone. It was pulling at my cheek and I could hardly talk or swallow. It was just a bad-looking thing and a bad-feeling thing, and it caused me a lot of pain.

This time I combined the therapy Dr. Schachter had me on with homeopathy. Basically, the therapies I used included eating organic foods and adding such things as laetrile, shark cartilage, homeopathic remedies, and a well-planned, well-thought-out vitamin and mineral program.

The bottom line is, it worked. Utilizing all the different therapies made the cancer shrink and vanish. My medical records show that it disappeared in two months and eleven days. That was little over a year ago. Any time I get an examination, everything is clean. I don't seem to have any sign of cancer. There is nothing like the alternative way of treating cancer.

Lucinda on Advanced Breast Cancer

I had severe breast cancer that metastasized to my ribs and throughout my whole spine. My prognosis was poor. Basically, I was told there was nothing they could do for me. Still, they wanted to try by putting me through the trauma of chemo and radiation, even though it wasn't going to cure me. It could only possibly prolong my life a little bit. I refused treatment, and they just sent me home to die with a box full of drugs.

Something inside of me said, "No, wait a minute, I choose not to do this. There's some other reason I'm supposed to be here." Through the grace of God, or the universe giving me another chance, I was put in contact with a clinic down in Mexico called Genesis West. I went down in a wheelchair on just about every drug you could possibly name. I was totally nonfunctional, mentally and physically.

In the clinic I received a wide variety of treatments. A few of them involved ozone therapy and hyperthermia. Of course, diet and supplementation to build the immune system were used. The whole basis of this is that the body is built to repair itself and that it has that capability.

I came back a total fighter. Now I'm walking, talking, and living my life completely and fully. I'm fighting every day, and I'm determined to beat this.

The change is nothing short of miraculous. In fact, the medical doctors are amazed. Of course, they don't want to admit it, but it's real concrete proof for them. I haven't gone in for any tests, like bone scan or MRI or anything like that yet, but they look at me and can see that I'm clear-eyed, walking, and functioning. Nobody can tell anything is wrong with me. Obviously, something I'm doing is working.

This experience has been a blessing for me. I want people to know that they have a lot more power and control within themselves than they know, and they need to learn that because there is always hope. You've got to always keep fighting if that's what you want.

Leslie on Metastatic Breast Cancer

I have been treated at Dr. Schachter's office for a little over a year. I came from Sloan-Kettering in Manhattan, where I was treated with radiation and chemotherapy. I was there for nine months. None of those treatments worked, and the cancer kept spreading. It finally spread to my liver, and I was given six months to live.

When I came to see Dr. Schachter, I was in pretty bad shape. When I started on his oral supplements, and later on his IV supplements, I started to get better. At the same time, I cut out dairy products and red meat and increased my intake of fresh fruits and vegetables. I made sure that I had no refined foods or sugar. If I did have something it would be from the organic food shelf rather than from a fast food chain. I started juicing and that gave me a tremendous lift in energy. My body was telling me that it was very happy. That was a turning point for me in knowing how important nutrition is in battling cancer.

I started to lose the cancer from my body. The tumor markers improved, and I started gaining weight. I had much more energy. At this point in time, my blood tests are back to normal. If you looked at me, you would not know I was a cancer patient.

What happened to me is amazing. I feel that it was a combination of the right treatments for me and a lot of prayer, creative visualization, and meditation. I continue to live that way now.

Ethyl on Metastatic Breast Cancer

I was originally diagnosed in November 1987. At that time, it spread to my bones and liver. I was on chemotherapy for two years, on and off, and was experiencing tremendous fatigue during and after chemotherapy. I had reactions where I had sores in my mouth, bleeding in my nose, and general malaise. Since starting direct ozone and vitamin drips, I have no more bleeding, no more sores, and no fatigue.

The last time I was in the hospital for chemotherapy, my doctor said to me, "We'll probably have to give you a transfusion." I replied, "I don't think you're right." He did some blood work and then told me that I was much stronger than he had thought I was.

I really feel a tremendous, tremendous difference. I can't wait until tomorrow to get my vitamin C drip because it is very healing for me. When I start getting ozone next week, I'm going to be a new person.

OXYGEN THERAPY

Richard on Prostate Cancer

Before discovering that I had prostate cancer, I had severe pains, especially during sexual relations. I was passing blood and had an awful time urinating. I went to see a specialist. After taking tests, he told me I had a solid cancer and that he needed to operate.

Fortunately, I learned through someone else about a doctor in Mexico. When I got to the clinic, my prostate count was 78. I began ozone treatments, and after three weeks, my count was down to 37. I continued treatments at home, and after six months, my count was down to zero. I continue using ozone to this very day. I take it in different ways. I have an ozone machine, and I use it when taking a bath, and I ozonate my drinking water as well. I use it a lot, because I feel if I don't, the cancer will come back.

Since my treatments, I feel better than I have felt in years. Now I can pass water without a problem. I can work and feel very good. I am more than pleased.

If it hadn't been for the ozone treatments, I wouldn't be here today, because that cancer would have had me. Surgery would have done no good.

Angelo on Colorectal Cancer with Metastases to the Liver

I was feeling tired every day and coming home to take a nap in the afternoon. That wasn't me. I had been a real active person all my life. My wife suggested that I take a blood test to see if anything was wrong. I did, and my doctor found that my blood was low. He suggested that I wait another week before taking another test, which I did. My blood was still low, so he suggested a colonoscopy. I went and had it done. The colonoscopy found a tumor in my colon. I had it operated on and taken out. The surgeon told me that he successfully removed it and that there was no more cancer there.

About three months later, I had a CT scan done that found spots on my liver. The cancer had metastasized on my liver. I received chemotherapy treatments for approximately six months. After the first set of treatments, another test was taken, which found that chemotherapy hadn't done any good. I continued with the chemotherapy for another three months. When that didn't help, the doctor said that there was nothing more he could do for me. I asked if I should continue with the chemo or just sit and die. He shrugged his shoulders, as if to say there was nothing more he could do for me. I asked the doctor how much time he thought I had and he said three to four months.

My son, who was there with me, had heard about a holistic program at Santa Monica Hospital utilizing ozone and vitamin therapy. He said I should take the treatments there, and I did. I received treatments for twenty-one days. They asked me to wait for eight weeks before having a CT scan. When I finally took the CT scan, the radiologist called my doctor and told him that he had never read a CT scan like mine before. It showed that the cancer cells in my liver had become capsulized. That prevented them from spreading.

The cancer cells have remained encapsulated, and I've been in remission for a year and a half. There is no question about it. The ozone treatment saved my life. In fact, I have so much faith in it now that I plan on going there every year and a half just to make sure that it stays that way.

Jane on Breast Cancer

I was diagnosed in 1989 with breast cancer, for which I had a modified radical mastectomy. I had numerous surgeries before that time as well. I wasn't really having any life at that point in time. I was a sick person waiting to die. They had cut out some of the cancer, but I wasn't well. A friend of mine finally advised me not to have any more of those treatments because they were killing me.

I had the book *Third Opinion*, which had something in it about Dr. Donsbach. I called Santa Monica Hospital and went down there. I was astounded by the humaneness of the Santa Monica Hospital. In other hospitals, I had some negative experiences where I felt totally robbed of all dignity and where I was treated like a specimen.

Santa Monica had a program that I could tolerate. I had decided that I was not going to have any more cutting, any more radiation, or any more chemo. There would be no more invasive procedures.

The first week I felt really, really sick because I was detoxifying from all the chemicals in my system. I had been on ten different medications for multiple problems. Besides cancer, I had ulcers, asthma, everything you could possibly imagine. The cancer had set off a systems reaction, and I was having problems in every part of my body.

After about the tenth day, I started to feel like getting out of bed. I began to participate in the therapies and started beach walks. I continued to get better and better.

I have been there six or seven times because I had some tumors in the other breast as well. I received ozone, hyperthermia, and thymus injections.

I don't have any tumors now. Most of all, I have a life. I work full time, and I play an active role in the lives of my granddaughter and daughters. I am able to go to church. I participate in library programs. I walk on the beach every day. I follow my program.

I learned things in the hospital that I need to be real careful with. Santa Monica Hospital will be the first place I go to if I begin developing symptoms. I don't think I will, though. I think I'm cured.

Charles on Prostate Cancer

I had a needle biopsy roughly a year ago, which indicated prostate cancer. I never believed in the orthodox approach and sought another method of treatment. Finally, I decided that I would go to Mexico and get treatment, which was not available in the United States. After doing a certain amount of research and checking with other people, I decided the Donsbach clinic in Rosarito Beach was the best place to go. I had been familiar with Dr. Donsbach for a number of years and felt that he offered the best options.

I feel that the treatment has been very satisfactory. At present my prostate has substantially improved. I'm not free of cancer yet, but there was not any promise that I would be that quickly. I am continuing outpatient care. But I feel it has most definitely made a difference. The PSA, for example, has dropped very substantially, which is probably the best measure of prostate cancer. I certainly feel a great deal better than when I first went to Rosarito Beach.

Gay on Colon Cancer

I was diagnosed with colon cancer in 1989. After they gave me eighteen months to live, I opted to find other alternatives and did so. I never received standard treatments even though they wanted to do surgery and chemotherapy.

Right now, I'm sitting on an IV of hydrogen peroxide with DMSO and all kinds of supplements and vitamins. That, along with a good diet and the help of a good friend, has gotten me this far. According to their predictions, I should have been dead in 1991 by the latest. In 1991, I made my second visit to the Hospital Santa Monica in Rosarito Beach.

Now I am in remission. When I am checked by the M.D.s, they are amazed. I have no more cancer in my colon. I have literally passed tumors through the rectum. The latest test showed that I have no tumors.

HIPPOCRATES HEALTH CENTER

Mike on Kidney Cancer

I'm a high school teacher from Los Angeles. In February of 1993, I had a kidney stone. After some X-rays and a CT scan, I was diagnosed with kidney cancer in my right kidney. I had two or three tumors. My doctor told me bluntly that if I didn't have a radical nephrectomy, which meant the extraction of all my lymph nodes underneath my arm all the way down to my hip, if I didn't take out my adrenal glands and kidney completely, and if I didn't have that operation by November of that year, I would be dead, no question about it. I told him that I wanted to get a second opinion, and he told me that it would be useless because it's cut and dried; there was no other thing that I could do.

My brother, Ronnie, was diagnosed as having cancer of the bone marrow by Sloan-Kettering and Johns Hopkins University. I called him to say that I had cancer, too. He told me to do what he did. He went to the Hippocrates Center and went on a fast. I went on a thirty-two-day water fast. Then I went on a seven-day juice fast. After that, I became a vegan. In other words, I didn't eat any meat, chicken, fish, or dairy products. I maintain that diet.

I go in for a CT scan every six months. The last one showed that the smallest tumor shrank a very small amount. I've had every kind of blood test and analysis that you can possibly think of. I just recently had one, and I sent it over to the Hippocrates Center because I'm going back there. They found that everything with my blood is 100 percent normal. I'm in great health.

The Hippocrates Center looks at you as a whole person. They don't threaten you; they just treat you like a human being. They use a natural diet. In other words, they don't heat anything up. Everything is a raw food and raw grains, slightly cooked.

I have maintained a phenomenal lifestyle. I'm active. I have three children. I'm not dead. I teach every day, and it's pretty hectic teaching in the *barrios* of Los Angeles. Yet I maintain a high activity in life. What can I tell you? Things look great; I'm alive, and I'm here.

George on Prostate Cancer

I went to a Hippocrates Health Center program for three weeks, about two years ago, and as a result of that, my prostate cancer went into remission. It was a program that consisted of organic, fresh, raw vegetables. It also consisted of green drinks, which were taken twice per day. In addition to that, there was a great deal of wheatgrass that I drank—also enemas. I did that for three weeks, and then I stayed on the program after I left the group. I went to the doctor about a week ago, and the doctor said that my cancer has disappeared; it is no longer there.

Additional Resources

Suggested Reading

- *Get Healthy Now*, by Gary Null
- *Be a Healthy Woman*, by Gary Null and Amy McDonald
- *The Complete Encyclopedia of Natural Healing*, by Gary Null
- *Fighting Cancer with Vitamins and Antioxidants*, by Kedar N. Prasad, Ph.D., and K. Che Prasad, M.S., M.D.
- *Flax Oil as a True Aid against Arthritis, Heart Infarction, Cancer, and Other Diseases*, by Dr. Johanna Budwig
- *Cancer—The Problem and the Solution*, by Dr. Johanna Budwig
- *The Cure for All Cancers*, by Dr. Hulda Clark
- *Natural Hygiene: Man's Pristine Way of Life*, by Dr. Herbert M. Shelton
- *Alternatives in Cancer Therapy: The Complete Guide to Non-traditional Treatments*, by Ross Pelton
- *Recalled by Life*, by Anthony J. Sattilaro
- *Alternative Medicine: The Definitive Guide* (2nd Edition), by Burton Goldberg Group
- *Cancer-Free: 30 Who Triumphed over Cancer Naturally*, by East West Foundation with Ann Fawcett and Cynthia Smith
- *Flood Your Body with Oxygen*, by Ed McCabe

- *The Cancer Prevention Diet: Michio Kushi's Macrobiotic Blueprint for the Prevention and Relief of Disease* by Michio Kushi with Alex Jack
- *The Macrobiotic Approach to Cancer: Towards Preventing and Controlling Cancer With Diet and Lifestyle*, by Michio Kushi
- *Cancer Diagnosis: What to Do Next*, by W. John Diamond
- *A Cancer Therapy: Results of Fifty Cases and the Cure of Advanced Cancer*, by Charlotte Gerson
- *Beating Cancer with Nutrition* (Revised), by Patrick Quillin and Noreen Quillin
- *How I Conquered Cancer Naturally*, by Eydie Mae and Chris Loeffler
- *Options: The Alternative Cancer Therapy Book*, by Richard Walters
- *Alive & Well: One Doctor's Experience with Nutrition in the Treatment of Cancer Patients*, by Philip E. Binzel
- *A Cancer Therapy: Results of Fifty Cases and the Cure of Advanced Cancer by Diet Therapy: A Summary of 30 Years of Clinical Experimentation*, by Max Gerson
- *Heinerman's Encyclopedia of Healing Juices*, by John Heinerman
- *The Breuss Cancer Cure: Advice for the Prevention and Natural Treatment of Cancer, Leukemia and Other Seemingly Incurable Diseases*, by Rudolf Breuss
- *Aveline Kushi's Complete Guide to Macrobiotic Cooking*, by Aveline Kushi
- *The Cure for All Advanced Cancers*, by Hulda Regehr Clark
- *The Cure for All Cancers: Including over 100 Case Histories of Persons Cured*, by Hulda Clark
- *One Answer to Cancer*, by William Donald Kelley
- *Health and Nutrition Secrets that Can Save Your Life*, by Russell L. Blaylock, M.D.

- *Cancer and Vitamin C: A Discussion of the Nature, Causes, Prevention, and Treatment of Cancer with Special Reference to the Value of Vitamin C*, by Ewan Cameron and Linus Pauling (Contributor)
- *Hyperbaric Oxygen Therapy*, by Morton Walker
- *When Hope Never Dies: One Woman's Remarkable Recovery from Cancer—And the Natural Program that Saved Her Life*, by Tom Monte
- *A Cancer Battle Plan: Six Strategies for Beating Cancer, from a Recovered "Hopeless Case,"* by Anne E. Frahm
- *The Cancer Cure that Worked: 50 Years of Suppression*, by Barry Lynes
- *Fats and Oils: The Complete Guide to Fats and Oils in Health and Nutrition*, by Udo Erasmus
- *Health Wars*, by Phillip Day
- *The Cancer Survival Cookbook: 200 Quick & Easy Recipes with Helpful Eating Hints,* by Donna L. Weihofen
- *Cancer—Why We're Still Dying to Know the Truth*, by Phillip Day
- *The Gerson Therapy: The Amazing Nutritional Program for Cancer and Other Illnesses*, by Charlotte Gerson
- *Dying to Look Good: The Disturbing Truth about What's Really in Your Cosmetics, Toiletries and Personal Care Products*, by Christine Hoza Farlow
- *Oxygen Healing Therapies: For Optimum Health & Vitality: Bio-Oxidative Therapies for Treating Immune Disorders, Candida, Cancer, Heart, Skin, Circulatory, and Other Modern Diseases*, by Nathaniel Altman
- *Introduction to Oxygen Therapies: Is This the Answer to Colds, Flu, AIDS, Cancer and Most Other Diseases*, by Ed McCabe
- *O2Xygen Therapies: A New Way of Approaching Disease,* by Ed McCabe

- *The Hippocrates Diet and Health Program*, by Ann Wigmore
- *The Burzynski Breakthrough*, by Thomas D. Elias
- *Ultimate Juicing: Delicious Recipes for over 125 of the Best Fruit and Vegetable Juice Combinations*, by Donna Pliner Rodnitzky
- *The Safe Shopper's Bible: A Consumer's Guide to Nontoxic Household Products*, by David Steinman and Samuel S. Epstein
- *The Complete Book of Enzyme Therapy*, by Anthony Cichoke
- *Cancer: Curing the Incurable without Surgery, Chemotherapy, or Radiation*, by William Donald Kelley
- *Gerson Diet Therapy for Women's Cancers: Breast Cancer, Ovarian Cancer, Cervical Cancer*, by Charlotte Gerson
- *Living Well Naturally*, by Anthony J. Sattilaro
- *Mind, Body, and Soul: A Guide to Living with Cancer*, by Nancy Hassett Dahm
- *Questioning Chemotherapy: A Critique of the Use of Toxic Drugs in the Treatment of Cancer*, by Ralph W. Moss
- *Cancer Therapy: The Independent Consumer's Guide to Non-toxic Treatment and Prevention*, by Ralph W. Moss
- *Censured for Curing Cancer: The American Experience of Dr. Max Gerson*, by Max Gerson
- *The Miraculous Diet: A New Era in Health & Well-Being: The Revolutionary Discoveries of Max Gerson, M.D.*, by Max Gerson
- *A Cancer Therapy: Results of Fifty Cases and the Cure of Advanced Cancer by Diet Therapy: A Summary of 30 Years of Clinical Experimentation*, by Max Gerson
- *World without Cancer: The Story of Vitamin B17*, by G. Edward Griffin
- *Your Face Never Lies: Introduction to Oriental Diagnosis*, by Michio Kushi

- *Beauty to Die For: The Cosmetic Consequence*, by Judi Vance
- *Drop-Dead Gorgeous: Protecting Yourself from the Hidden Dangers of Cosmetics*, by Kim Erickson
- *Hydrogen Peroxide: Medical Miracle*, by William Campbell Douglass
- *Healing Cancer*, by Michio Kushi
- *A Consumer's Dictionary of Cosmetic Ingredients*, by Ruth Winter
- *The Miracle of Fasting: Proven throughout History for Physical, Mental and Spiritual Rejuvenation*, by Paul C. Bragg and Patricia Bragg
- *Return to Wholeness: Embracing Body, Mind, and Spirit in the Face of Cancer*, by Deepak Chopra
- *Tomato Power: Lycopene: The Miracle Nutrient that Can Prevent Aging, Heart Disease and Cancer*, by James F. Balch
- *How to Prevent Breast Cancer*, by Ross Pelton
- *What to Eat if You Have Cancer*, by Daniella Chace and Maureen Keane
- *The Prostate: A Guide for Men and the Women Who Love Them*, Patrick C. Walsh, M.D., and Janet Farrar Worthington
- *How to Fight Cancer & Win*, by William L. Fischer
- *The Juicing Bible*, by Pat Crocker and Susan Eagles
- *Safer Medicine*, by Mayer Eisenstein
- *The Cancer Industry: The Classic Exposé on the Cancer Establishment*, by Ralph W. Moss
- *Coping with Cancer: How to Prevent and Treat Cancer with Vitamins, Minerals, and Diet*, by Morton Walker
- *Dr. Max Gerson: Healing the Hopeless*, by Max Gerson
- *My Beautiful Life: How Macrobiotics Brought Me from Cancer to Radiant Health*, by Milenka Dobic
- *The Shocking Truth about Water*, by Paul C. Bragg and Patricia Bragg

- *Apple Cider Vinegar—Miracle Health System*, by Paul C. Bragg and Patricia Bragg
- *The What to Eat if You Have Cancer Cookbook*, by Daniella Chace and Maureen Keane
- *Healing outside the Margins: The Survivor's Guide to Integrative Cancer Care*, by Carole O'Toole and Carolyn B. Hendricks, M.D.

Suggested Documentaries

- *Preventing and Reversing Cancer Naturally,* by Gary Null
- *Burzynski: The Movie,* by Eric Mercola
- *Cut, Poison, Burn*, by Wayne Chesler
- *Pink Ribbons, Inc.*, by Lea Pool
- *Healing Cancer*, by Mike Anderson
- *The Beautiful Truth*, by Steve Kroschel
- *Dying to Have Known*, by Steve Kroschel
- *The Gerson Miracle*, by Steve Kroschel

About the Author

An internationally renowned expert in the field of health and nutrition, Gary Null, Ph.D is the author of over 70 best-selling books on healthy living and the director of over 100 critically acclaimed full-feature documentary films on natural health, self-empowerment and the environment. He is the host of "The Gary Null Show", the country's longest running nationally syndicated health radio talk show which can be heard daily on ProgressiveRadioNetwork.com.

Endnotes

[1] "41 percent of Americans will get cancer." UPI.com. http://www.upi.com/Health_News/2010/05/06/41-percent-of-Americans-will-get-cancer/UPI-75711273192042/ (accessed March 2, 2012).

[2] "Why We Are Still Losing the Winnable War Against Cancer." World-Wire http://world-wire.com/2011/12/09/why-we-are-still-losing-the-winnable-war-against-cancer/ (accessed January 16, 2012).

[3] Epstein, Samuel S. *National Cancer Institute and American Cancer Society: Criminal Indifference to Cancer Prevention and Conflicts of Interest.* Self-Published Manuscript. United States: Xlibris Corporation, 2011.

[4] Ibid.

[5] Ibid.

[6] Pierce, Tanya Harter. *Outsmart Your Cancer: Alternative Non-toxic Treatments that Work.* 2nd ed. Stateline, NV: Thoughtworks Publishing, 2009.

[7] "How the Losing Cancer War Is Being Spun Warns Samuel S. Epstein, M.D." PR Newswire. http://www.prnewswire.com/news-releases/how-the-losing-cancer-war-is-being-spun-warns-samuel-s-epstein-md-and-quentin-d-young-md-71761482.html (accessed January 16, 2012).

[8] "The NCI Annual Fact Book" Office of Budget and Finance. http://obf.cancer.gov/financial/factbook.htm (accessed August 21, 2013).

[9] Epstein, Samuel S. *National Cancer Institute and American Cancer Society: Criminal Indifference to Cancer Prevention and Conflicts of Interest.* Self-Published Manuscript. United States: Xlibris Corporation, 2011.

[10] "FY 2013 Budget" National Cancer Institute http://obf.cancer.gov/financial/attachments/2013cj.pdf (accessed August 20, 2013)

[11] "Medical Experts Prescribe Legislation to Help Prevent Cancer." world-wire.com. http://world-wire.com/news/0906150001.html (accessed January 23, 2012).

[12] Ibid.

[13] Ho, Dr. Mae-Wan. "Cancer:An Epigenetic Disease." The Institute of Science in Society. http://www.i-sis.org.uk/Cancer_an_Epigenetic_Disease.php (accessed April 5, 2012).

[14] Rubin, Harry, and Bryan Ellison. "Individual Transforming Events in Long-Term Cell Culture of NIH 3T3 Cells as Products of Epigenetic Induction." *Cancer Research* 52 (1992). http://cancerres.aacrjournals.org/content/52/3/667.full.pdf (accessed April 2, 2012).

[15] Ho, Dr. Mae-Wan. "Cancer:An Epigenetic Disease." The Institute of Science in Society. http://www.i-sis.org.uk/Cancer_an_Epigenetic_Disease.php (accessed April 5, 2012).

[16] Ibid.

[17] Null, Gary, and Robert Houston. "The Great Cancer Fraud." Available at Legacy Tobacco Documents Library. Reprinted from *Penthouse*, 1979. http://legacy.library.ucsf.edu/tid/ter51e 00;jsessionid=34B2F322366104BD923E3AB60D6430A8 (accessed March 19, 2012).

[18] Epstein, Samuel. "Samuel S. Epstein: The American Cancer Society Trivializes Cancer Risks: Blatant Conflicts of Interest." The Huffington Post. http://www.huffingtonpost.com/samuel-s-epstein/the-american-cancer-socie_b_568292.html (accessed January 23, 2012).

[19] Ibid.

[20] Ibid.

[21] Epstein, Samuel S. *National Cancer Institute and American Cancer Society: Criminal Indifference to Cancer Prevention and Conflicts of Interest*. Self-Published Manuscript. United States: Xlibris Corporation, 2011(accessed March 19, 2012).

[22] Ibid.

[23] Ibid.

[24] Ibid.

[25] "Recombinant Bovine Growth Hormone." American Cancer Society. http://www.cancer.org/cancer/cancercauses/othercarcinogens/athome/recombinant-bovine-growth-hormone (accessed January 31, 2012).

[26] Israel, Brett. "How Many Cancers Are Caused by the Environment?" *Scientific American*, May 21, 2010. http://www.scientificamerican.com/article.cfm?id=how-many-cancers-are-caused-by-the-environment (accessed February 8, 2012).

[27] Davis D., *The Secret History of the War on Cancer*, Basic Books, New York, 2009.

[28] Sanet, Jonathan M, and Frank Speizer. "Sir Richard Doll, 1912–2005." *American Journal of Epidemiology* 164, no. 1 (2006): 95-100. http://aje.oxfordjournals.org/content/164/1/95.full (accessed March 13, 2012).

[29] "American Cancer Society: More Interested in Accumulating Wealth than Saving Lives." www.wnho.net/acs.pdf (accessed January 30, 2012).

[30] Epstein, Samuel S. "The Stop Cancer Before Before it Starts Campaign: How to Win the Losing War Against Cancer." Preventcancer.com. http://www.preventcancer.com/press/pdfs/Stop_Cancer_Book.pdf (accessed August 13, 2013).

[31] Boseley, Sarah. "Renowned Cancer Scientist Was Paid by Chemical Firm for 20 Years." *The Guardian*. http://www.guardian.co.uk/science/2006/dec/08/smoking.frontpagenews (accessed February 14, 2012).

[32] Ibid.

[33] Ibid.

[34] Ibid.

[35] Ibid.

[36] Epstein, Samuel S. "The Stop Cancer Before Before it Starts Campaign: How to Win the Losing War Against Cancer." Preventcancer.com. http://www.preventcancer.com/press/pdfs/Stop_Cancer_Book.pdf (accessed August 13, 2013).

[37] Davis D., *The Secret History of the War on Cancer*, Basic Books, New York, 2009.

[38] Ibid.

[39] Epstein, Samuel S. "The Stop Cancer Before Before it Starts Campaign: How to Win the Losing War Against Cancer." Preventcancer.com. http://www.preventcancer.com/press/pdfs/Stop_Cancer_Book.pdf (accessed August 13, 2013).

[40] Null, Gary, and Robert Houston. "Legacy Tobacco Documents Library: The Great Cancer Fraud." Legacy Tobacco Documents Library. http://legacy.library.ucsf.edu/tid/ter51e00;jsessionid=34B2F322366104BD923E3AB60D6430A8 (accessed March 19, 2012).

[41] Ausubel, Ken. *When Healing Becomes a Crime: The Amazing Story of the Hoxsey Cancer Clinics and the Return of Alternative Therapies.* Rochester, VT: Healing Arts Press, 2000.

[42] American Cancer Society. "The Position of the American Cancer Society Regarding Tobacco and Lung Cancer [Historical Overview of ACS Fight against Tobacco Use and Possible Link to Lung Cancer]." Available at Tobacco Documents Online http://webcache.googleusercontent.com/search?q=cache:10MJIMUK_1kJ:tobaccodocuments.org/ctr/11316540-6570.html%3Fstart_page%3D11%26end_page%3D12+&cd=1&hl=en&ct=clnk&gl=us (accessed January 25, 2012).

[43] Davis, Devra Lee. *The Secret History of the War on Cancer.* New York: BasicBooks, 2007.

[44] Epstein, Samuel. "Samuel S. Epstein: The American Cancer Society Trivializes Cancer Risks: Blatant Conflicts of Interest." The Huffington Post. http://www.huffingtonpost.com/samuel-s-epstein/the-american-cancer-socie_b_568292.html (accessed January 23, 2012).

[45] Epstein, Samuel. "The American Cancer Society: The World's Wealthiest "Nonprofit" Institution." Archive.IS. http://archive.is/zS9Do (accessed November 14, 2013).

[46] Ibid.

[47] Ibid.

[48] "Charity Navigator Rating—American Cancer Society." Charity Navigator. http://www.charitynavigator.org/index.cfm?bay=search.summary&orgid=6495 (accessed January 19, 2012).

[49] Ibid.

[50] Ibid.

[51] Epstein, Samuel S. *National Cancer Institute and American Cancer Society: Criminal Indifference to Cancer Prevention and Conflicts of Interest.* Self-Published Manuscript. United States: Xlibris Corporation, 2011.

[52] Ibid.

[53] Ibid.

[54] "Why We Are Still Losing the Winnable War against Cancer." World-Wire. http://world-wire.com/2011/12/09/why-we-are-still-losing-the-winnable-war-against-cancer/ (accessed March 16, 2012).

[55] Marchione, Marilynn. "Taxol may be ineffective for many cancer patients." Deseret News, November 10, 2007. http://www.deseretnews.com/article/695217600/Taxol-may-be-ineffective-for-many-cancer-patients.html?pg=all (accessed March 6, 2013).

[56] Ibid.

[57] Cummins, Ronnie, Janette Sherman, Quentin Young, and Samuel Epstein. "Why We Are Still Losing the Winnable War Against Cancer." WorldWire. http://world-wire.com/2011/12/09/why-we-are-still-losing-the-winnable-war-against-cancer/ (accessed November 14, 2013).

[58] Epstein, Samuel S. *National Cancer Institute and American Cancer Society: Criminal Indifference to Cancer Prevention and Conflicts of Interest.* Self-Published Manuscript. United States: Xlibris Corporation, 2011.

[59] Epstein, Samuel S. *Cancer-gate: how to win the losing cancer war.* Amityville, N.Y.: Baywood Pub., 2005.

[60] Cummins, Ronnie, Janette Sherman, Quentin Young, and Samuel Epstein. "Why We Are Still Losing the Winnable War Against Cancer." WorldWire. http://world-wire.com/2011/12/09/why-we-are-still-losing-the-winnable-war-against-cancer/ (accessed November 14, 2013).

[61] Epstein, Samuel S. "Asleep at the Wheel of the War on Cancer." Physicians for Social Responsibility. http://www.psr.org/environment-and-health/environmental-health-policy-institute/responses/asleep-at-the-wheel-of-the-war-on-cancer.html (accessed March 19, 2012).

[62] "Review finds conflicts of interest in many cancer studie." e! Science News. http://esciencenews.com/articles/2009/05/11/review.finds.conflicts.interest.many.cancer.studies (accessed March 16, 2012).

[63] Epstein, Samuel S. *National Cancer Institute and American Cancer Society: Criminal Indifference to Cancer Prevention and Conflicts of Interest.*Self-Published Manuscript. United States: Xlibris Corporation, 2011.

[64] Moss, Ralph." The Ralph Moss Story." www.whale.to/cancer/ralph_moss_story.html (accessed March 5, 2012).

[65] Ibid.

[66] Ibid.

[67] Ibid.

[68] "Memorial Sloan-Kettering Cancer Center." SourceWatch. http://www.sourcewatch.org/index.php?title=Memorial_Sloan-Kettering_Cancer_Center#cite_note-14 (accessed March 27, 2012).

[69] "Paul Marks: Executive Profile & Biography." Businessweek. http://investing.businessweek.com/research/stocks/people/person.asp?personId=83425075&ticker=EVN:AU&previousCapId=9376903&previousTitle=OCEANAGOLD%20CORP-CDI (accessed March 27, 2012).

[70] "Board of Directors." Merck. http://www.merck.com/about/leadership/board-of-directors/home.html (accessed March 6, 2012).

[71] Cone, Maria. "President's Cancer Panel: Environmentally Caused Cancers Are 'Grossly Underestimated' and 'Needlessly Devastate American Lives'." Environmental Health News. http://www.environmentalhealthnews.org/ehs/news/presidents-cancer-panel (accessed February 15, 2012).

[72] Epstein, Samuel. "President's Cancer Panel Warns of Toxic Effects of BPA." The Huffington Post. http://www.huffingtonpost.com/samuel-s-epstein/presidents-cancer-panel-w_b_566541.html (accessed November 14, 2013)

[73] Epstein, Samuel. "Samuel S. Epstein: President's Cancer Panel Warns of Toxic Effects of BPA." The Huffington Post. http://www.huffingtonpost.com/samuel-s-epstein/presidents-cancer-panel-w_b_566541.html (accessed March 9, 2012).

[74] "Update on Bisphenol A for Use in Food Contact Applications: January 2010." Food Processing Suppliers Association (FPSA) I. http://www.fpsa.org/update-bisphenol-use-food-contact-applications-january-2010 (accessed November 14, 2013).

[75] Carollo, Kim. "FDA Rejects Ban on BPA—." ABCNews. http://abcnews.go.com/Health/fda-rejects-ban-bpa/story?id=16038492 (accessed April 9, 2012).

[76] Silverstein, Amy. "Is Susan G. Komen Denying the BPA-Breast Cancer Link? Mother Jones. http://motherjones.com/environment/2011/09/breast-cancer-komen-bpa (accessed March 9, 2012).

[77] Ibid.

[78] Ibid.

[79] "Reducing Environmental Cancer Risk: What We Can Do Now." National Cancer Institute. http://deainfo.nci.nih.gov/advisory/pcp/annualReports/pcp08-09rpt/PCP_Report_08-09_508.pdf (accessed August 12, 2013).

[80] Harris, Gardiner. "Formaldehyde Is Added to List of Carcinogens—." *New York Times.* http://www.nytimes.com/2011/06/11/health/11cancer.html (accessed March 9, 2012).

[81] Epstein, Samuel. "Milk: America's Health Problem." American Nutrition Association. http://americannutritionassociation.org/toolsandresources/milk-

america%C3%A2%E2%82%AC%E2%84%A2s-health-problem (accessed November 14, 2013).

82 "AICR Statement: Hot Dogs and Cancer Risk." Medical News Today. http://www.medical-newstoday.com/releases/158507.php (accessed March 12, 2012).

83 "The 'Dirty Dozen' Consumer Products." Cancer Prevention Coalition. http://www.preventcancer.com/consumers/general/dirty_dozen.htm (accessed February 15, 2012).

84 Moore, Nancy. "Cancer-Causing Foods: 3 Culprits and 6 Top Foods." Natural Healing, Natural Health. http://www.natural-healing-health.com/Cancer-Causing-Foods.html (accessed March 12, 2012).

85 "Annual Report to the Nation Shows Continuing Decline in Cancer Mortality." *JNCI*. http://jnci.oxfordjournals.org/content/103/9/NP.1 (accessed February 15, 2012).

86 "CSPI Says Food Dyes Pose Rainbow of Risks." Center for Science in the Public Interest. http://www.cspinet.org/new/201006291.html (accessed February 15, 2012).

87 Bracy, Kate. "Toxic Beauty: The Ugly Truth about Cosmetics." *American Nurse Today* 6, no. 5 (2011). http://www.americannursetoday.com/article.aspx?id=7820&fid=7770 (accessed March 5, 2012).

88 Ibid.

89 Ibid.

90 "The 'Dirty Dozen' Ingredients Investigated in the David Suzuki Foundation Survey of Chemicals in Cosmetics." www.davidsuzuki.org. http://www.davidsuzuki.org/issues/downloads/Dirty-dozen-backgrounder.pdf (accessed March 6, 2012).

91 Ibid.

92 "FDA: Some Chicken May Have Small Amount of Arsenic" phillyBurbs.com. http://usatoday30.usatoday.com/money/industries/food/2011-06-08-fda-chicken-arsenic_n.htm (accessed March 12, 2012).

93 Adams, Mike. "FDA Finally Admits Chicken Meat Contains Cancer-Causing Arsenic (but Keep Eating It, Yo!)." Natural Health News. http://www.naturalnews.com/032659_arsenic_chicken.html (accessed March 12, 2012).

94 "FDA: Some Chicken May Have Small Amount of Arsenic." phillyBurbs.com. http://usatoday30.usatoday.com/money/industries/food/2011-06-08-fda-chicken-arsenic_n.htm (accessed March 12, 2012).

95 "Questions and Answers Regarding 3-Nitro(Roxarsone)." U.S. Food and Drug Administration. http://www.fda.gov/AnimalVeterinary/SafetyHealth/ProductSafetyInformation/ucm258313.htm (accessed March 13, 2012).

96 Ibid.

97 Ibid.

98 Smith, Jeffrey. "Jeffrey Smith: Obama's Team Includes Dangerous Biotech 'Yes Men.'" The Huffington Post. http://www.huffingtonpost.com/jeffrey-smith/obamas-team-includes-dang_b_147188.html (accessed March 13, 2012).

99 Null, Gary, and Jeremy Stillman." The Dirty Dozen Drugs" Scribd. http://www.scribd.com/doc/70552555/The-Dirty-Dozen-Drugs-by-Gary-Null-Ph-D (accessed March 12, 2012).

100 Ibid.

101 "CFR—Code of Federal Regulations Title 21." FDA.gov. www.accessdata.fda.gov/scripts/cdrh/cfdocs/cfcfr/CFRSearch.cfm?fr=558.369 (accessed February 28, 2012).

102 Ibid.

103 Ibid.

[104] "Environmental Health Perspectives: Seafood Contamination after the BP Gulf Oil Spill and Risks to Vulnerable Populations: A Critique of the FDA Risk Assessment." Environmental Health Perspectives. http://ehp03.niehs.nih.gov/article/info%3Adoi%2F10.1289%2Fehp.11 03695#top (accessed March 14, 2012).

[105] Ibid.

[106] Ibid.

[107] Jacobson, Brad. "FDA OK's High Levels of Dangerous Carcinogens in Seafood." Reader Supported News. http://readersupportednews.org/news-section2/313-17/8994-fda-oks-high-levels-of-dangerous-carcinogens-in-seafood (accessed March 14, 2012).

[108] "Lobbying Spending Database, Food & Drug Administration, 2011." OpenSecrets.org. http://www.opensecrets.org/lobby/agencysum.php?id=135 (accessed March 15, 2012).

[109] Parker-Pope, Tara. "Mammogram's Role as Savior Is Tested." *The New York Times*, October 24, 2011. http://well.blogs.nytimes.com/2011/10/24/mammograms-role-as-savior-is-tested/ (accessed November 14, 2013).

[110] Kruk, J, and H Aboulenein. "Psychological Stress and The Risk Of Breast Cancer: A Case Control Study." *Cancer Detection and Prevention* 28, no. 6 (2004): 399-408.

[111] Prate, Dawn. "Mammograms Cause Breast Cancer (And Other Cancer Facts You Probably Never Knew." *Natural News*. http://www.naturalnews.com/010886.html (accessed Oct 1, 2013).

[112] Kawa, Lucas. "Regular Doctor's Check-Ups are a Big Waste of Money." *Business Insider*. http://www.businessinsider.com/check-ups-dont-improve-health-outcomes-2013-1 (accessed Oct 1, 2013).

[113] Welch, HG, and BA Frankel. "Likelihood that a Woman with Screen-Detected Breast Cancer Has Had Her 'Life Saved' by That Screening." *Arch Intern Med* 171, no. 22 (2011): 2043-6.

[114] Wright, C.J., and C.B. Mueller. "Screening Mammography And Public Health Policy: The Need For Perspective." The Lancet346, no. 8966 (1995): 29-32.

[115] Welch, H. G., S. Woloshin, and L. M. Schwartz. "The Sea Of Uncertainty Surrounding Ductal Carcinoma In Situ–The Price Of Screening Mammography."*JNCI Journal of the National Cancer Institute* 100, no. 4 (2008): 228-229.

[116] "Thermography Is a Safe Alternative to Mammography." Natural Health News. http://www.naturalnews.com/033586_thermography_mammography.html (accessed February 2, 2012).

[117] Ibid.

[118] Epstein, Samuel. "Corporate Sponsors Control Mammography Industry Warns Cancer Prevention Coalition." World-Wire. http://world-wire.com/2011/10/21/corporate-sponsors-control-mammography-industry-warns-cancer-prevention-coalition (accessed February 3, 2012).

[119] Gale, Jason. "Prostate Exam Deaths From 'Superbugs' Spur Inquiry Into Cancer Tests." Bloomberg. http://www.bloomberg.com/news/2011-05-05/prostate-exam-deaths-tied-to-superbug-ills-spur-cancer-test-inquiries.html (accessed February 1, 2012).

[120] Ibid.

[121] Gordon, Serena. "Prostate Biopsies Can Raise Risk of Hospitalization." USATODAY.com. http://yourlife.usatoday.com/health/medical/menshealth/story/2011-09-23/Prostate-biopsies-can-raise-risk-of-hospitalization-in-older-men/50528990/1 (accessed February 1, 2012).

[122] Sandblom et al. "Randomised Prostate Cancer Screening Trial: 20-Year Follow-Up." *British Medical Journal*1;342:d1539 (2011). http://www.bmj.com/content/342/bmj.d1539 (accessed January 18, 2012).

[123] Schröder et al. "Screening and Prostate-Cancer Mortality in a Randomized European Study." *The New England Journal of Medicine* 360:1320-1328 (2009). http://www.nejm.org/doi/full/10.1056/NEJMoa0810084 (accessed January 23, 2012).

[124] Ibid.

[125] Marchione, Marilynn. "Setback Reported in Research into Cancer Treatment." Yahoo! News. http://news.yahoo.com/setback-reported-research-cancer-treatment-222634604.html (accessed November 14, 2013).

[126] University of Michigan Comprehensive Cancer Center. "50 is the Golden Age to Begin Routine Colonoscopies" http://www.med.umich.edu/cancer/news/colonoscopy05.shtml (accessed 8/4/13)

[127] U.S. Multisociety Task Force on Colorectal Cancer et. al. "Colorectal Cancer Screening and Surveillance" https://www.med.upenn.edu/gastro/documents/AGAtechnicalreviewcolorectalcancerscreening.pdf (accessed 8/20/13)

[128] W.S. Atkin& B.P. Saunders. "SurveillanceGuidelinesAfter Removal of Colorectal Adenomatous Polyps" http://gut.bmj.com/content/51/suppl_5/v6.full.pdf (accessed 8/20/13)

[129] WebMD. "Colonoscopy" http://www.webmd.com/colorectal-cancer/colonoscopy-16695 (accessed 8/0/13)

[130] UK Department for Work and Pensions "Tests for Bowel Cancer Including Rectal Cancer" http://webarchive.nationalarchives.gov.uk/+/http://www.dwp.gov.uk/publications/specialist-guides/medical-conditions/a-z-of-medical-conditions/bowel-cancer/tests-bowel-cancer.shtml(accessed 8/20/13)

[131] Levin, TR et. al. "Complications of Colonoscopy in an Integrated Health Care Delivery System." Ann Intern Med 145, no. 12 (2006): 880-6.

[132] Johns Hopkins Medicine. "Colonoscopy" http://www.hopkinsmedicine.org/healthlibrary/test_procedures/gastroenterology/colonoscopy_92,P07693/ (accessed 8/20/13)

[133] Rabenecket et al. "Bleeding and perforation after outpatient colonoscopy and their risk factors in usual clinical practice" http://www.ncbi.nlm.nih.gov/pubmed/18938166 (accessed 8/20/13)

[134] Lawrence B. Cohen, MD, Faculty, David M. Kastenberg, MD, Faculty, David B. Mount, MD, Faculty, and Alan V. Safdi, MD, Faculty "Current Issues in Optimal Bowel Preparation." *Gastroenterol Hepatol* 5 (2009): 3-11.

[135] "Grade Definitions After May 2007." (USPSTF). http://www.uspreventiveservicestaskforce.org/uspstf/gradespost.htm#crec (accessed November 14, 2013).

[136] Tanner, Lindsay. "Study: Many Elderly Get Colon Screening Too Often." The Washingtion Times. http://www.washingtontimes.com/news/2011/may/9/study-many-elderly-get-colon-screening-too-often/?page=all (accessed November 14, 2013).

[137] "Study: Many Elderly Get Colon Screening Too Often." Yahoo! Health. http://neurotalk.psychcentral.com/thread149881.html (accessed 2/2/12)

[138] Sharp, Kathleen. *Blood Feud: The Man Who Blew the Whistle on One of the Deadliest Prescription Drugs Ever.* New York: Dutton, 2011.

[139] Ibid.

[140] Reinberg, Steven. "Anemia Drugs May Raise Death Risk in Cancer Patients." Health.com. http://news.health.com/2009/05/01/anemia-drugs-may-raise-death-risk-cancer-patients/ (accessed March 1, 2012).

[141] Harris, Gardiner. "FDA Urges Doctors to Cut Back on Anemia Drugs." *New York Times.* http://www.nytimes.com/2011/06/25/health/policy/25drug.html?_r=2&partner=rss&emc=rss (accessed February 29, 2012).

142 Ibid.

143 Reinberg, Steven. "Anemia Drugs May Raise Death Risk in Cancer Patients." Health. com. http://news.health.com/2009/05/01/anemia-drugs-may-raise-death-risk-cancer-patients/ (accessed February 29, 2012).

144 Harris, Gardiner. "FDA Urges Doctors to Cut Back on Anemia Drugs." *New York Times*. http://www.nytimes.com/2011/06/25/health/policy/25drug.html?_r=2&partner=rss&emc=rss (accessed February 29, 2012).

145 Marchione, Marilynn. "USA TODAY." USATODAY.COM. http://usatoday30.usatoday.com/news/health/story/health/story/2012-03-07/Setback-reported-in-research-into-cancer-treatment/53402208/1 (accessed November 14, 2013).

146 Ibid.

147 "Questions about Chemotherapy." American Cancer Society. http://www.cancer.org/Treatment/TreatmentsandSideEffects/TreatmentTypes/Chemotherapy/WhatItIsHowItHelps/chemo-what-it-is-questions-about-chemo (accessed March 9, 2012).

148 Moss, Ralph W. *Questioning Chemotherapy*. Brooklyn, NY: Equinox Press, 1995.

149 Ibid.

150 "The Contribution of Cytotoxic Chemotherapy to 5-Year Survival in Adult Malignancies." *ClinOncol (R CollRadiol)*, 2004. http://www.ncbi.nlm.nih.gov/pubmed/15630849 (accessed March 5, 2012).

151 Reference # 151 - Chow, Reuben. "Study Reveals Chemotherapy Hastened or Caused Deaths of Many." NaturalNews. http://www.naturalnews.com/025499_cancer_chemotherapy_treatment.html (accessed November 15, 2013).

153 Ibid.

154 "The Risk of Developing Uterine Sarcoma after Tamoxifen Use." *International Journal of Gynecological Cancer*, 2007." Wiley Online Library. http://onlinelibrary.wiley.com/doi/10.1111/j.1525-1438.2007.01025.x/abstract (accessed March 6, 2012).

155 Smith, Carol. "Lifesaving Drugs May Be Killing Health Workers." The Seattle Times. http://seattletimes.nwsource.com/html/localnews/2012327665_chemo11.html (accessed February 28, 2012).

156 "Law Would Level the Playing Field for Chemotherapy Pills." RVANews. http://rvanews.com/news/law-would-level-the-playing-field-for-chemotherapy-pills/57342 (accessed March 5, 2012).

157 Marchione, Marilynn. "Provenge, Cancer Drug, Costs $93,000: Sky-High Drug Prices Impact Life-Or-Death Decisions." The Huffington Post. http://www.huffingtonpost.com/2010/09/26/provenge-cancer-drug-cost_n_739722.html (accessed March 6, 2012).

158 "Law Would Level the Playing Field for Chemotherapy Pills." RVANews. http://rvanews.com/news/law-would-level-the-playing-field-for-chemotherapy-pills/57342 (accessed March 5, 2012).

159 Ibid.

160 Edwards, Jim. "Why a $93,000 Cancer Drug Can't Shake Off Rumors It Doesn't Work." CBS News. http://www.cbsnews.com/8301-505123_162-42845241/why-a-93000-cancer-drug-cant-shake-off-rumors-it-doesnt-work/?tag=bnetdomain (accessed March 6, 2012).

161 Edwards, Jim. "Dendreon CEO Dumped $1M in Stock Before Withdrawing Revenue Guidance." CBS News. http://www.cbsnews.com/8301-505123_162-42849362/dendreon-ceo-dumped-1m-in-stock-before-withdrawing-revenue-guidance/ (accessed March 6, 2012).

162 NCEPOD—SACT: For Better, for Worse? Report (2008)." National Confidential Enquiry into Patient Outcome and Death. http://www.ncepod.org.uk/2008sact.htm (accessed March 5, 2012).

[163] Pollack, Andrew. "Heated, Harrowing Chemotherapy Bath May Be Only Hope for Some." *New York Times*. http://www.nytimes.com/2011/08/12/business/heated-chemotherapy-bath-may-be-only-hope-for-some-cancer-patients.html (accessed February 28, 2012).

[164] Ibid.

[165] Ausubel, Ken. *When Healing Becomes a Crime: The Amazing Story of the HoxseyCancer Clinics and the Return of Alternative Therapies*. Rochester, VT: Healing Arts Press, 2000.

[166] "Self-Seeding of Cancer Cells May Play a Critical Role in Tumor Progression | Memorial Sloan-Kettering Cancer Center." Memorial Sloan-Kettering Cancer Center. http://www.mskcc.org/news/press/self-seeding-cells-may-play-critical-role-tumor-progression (accessed March 2, 2012).

[167] Grady, Denise. "Repeat Breast Cancer Surgery Guidelines Found Unclear." *New York Times*. http://www.nytimes.com/2012/02/01/health/repeat-breast-cancer-surgery-guidelines-found-unclear.html?_r=1&scp=2&sq=breast percent20cancer&st=cse (accessed February 28, 2012).

[168] "Arch Surg—Abstract: Unnecessary Axillary Surgery for Patients With Node-Negative Breast Cancer Undergoing Total Mastectomy, September 2011, Olaya et al. 146 (9): 1029." *Archives of Surgery*. http://archsurg.ama-assn.org/cgi/content/abstract/146/9/1029 (accessed March 2, 2012).

[169] Grady, Denise. "Lymph Node Surgery for Breast Cancer Not Always Needed, Study Says." *New York Times*. http://www.nytimes.com/2011/02/09/health/research/09breast.html?pagewanted=all (accessed March 2, 2012).

[170] Ibid.

[171] Griffin, G. Edward. *World without Cancer*. Westlake Village, CA: American Media, 2000.

[172] Faloon, William. "Cancer Establishment Hides Radiation Side Effects." Life Extension. http://www.lef.org/magazine/mag2011/dec2011_Cancer-Establishment-Hides-Radiation-Side-Effects_01.htm (accessed March 7, 2012).

[173] Ibid.

[174] Ibid.

[175] "Radiation of Left Breast during Cancer Treatment Causes Coronary Artery Disease." Natural Health News. http://www.naturalnews.com/019989_conventional_cancer_treatments_radiation_therapy.html (accessed March 7, 2012).

[176] Gutierrez, David. "Radiation Treatment for Cancer Causes Diabetes in Children." Natural Health News. http://www.naturalnews.com/028032_radiation_therapy_diabetes.html (accessed March 7, 2012).

[177] Ibid.

[178] Samadi, David. "New Dangers of Radiation Therapy Exposed." Fox News. http://www.foxnews.com/health/2011/01/04/new-dangers-radiation-therapy-exposed/ (accessed November 25, 2013).

[179] Ibid.

[180] Bogdanich, Walt. "The Radiation Boom—Radiation Offers New Cures, and Ways to Do Harm." *New York Times*. http://www.nytimes.com/2010/01/24/health/24radiation.html?ref=health (accessed March 7, 2012).

[181] Gripp, Stephan, Sibylle Mjartan, Edwin Boelke, and Reinhardt Willers. "Palliative Radiotherapy Tailored To Life Expectancy In End-stage Cancer Patients." Cancer116, no. 13 (2010): 3251-3256.

[182] Ibid.

[183] Ibid.

[184] Smith, BD, et. al. "Adoption of intensity-modulated radiation therapy for breast cancer in the United States." *J Natl Cancer Inst* 103, no. 10 (2011): 798-809.

[185] "NCI Cancer Bulletin for May 3, 2011." National Cancer Institute. http://www.cancer.gov/ncicancerbulletin/050311/page3 (accessed March 8, 2012).

[186] Nguyen, Paul, et al. "Cost Implications of the Rapid Adoption of Newer Technologies for Treating Prostate Cancer." *Journal of Clinical Oncology* 31, no. 1217 (2011): 1-11.

[187] Ibid.

[188] Null, Gary, and Robert Houston. "Legacy Tobacco Documents Library: The Great Cancer Fraud" Legacy Tobacco Documents Library . http://legacy.library.ucsf.edu/tid/ter51e00;jsessionid=34B2F322366104BD923E3AB60D6430A8 (accessed March 19, 2012).

[189] Ibid.

[190] "Gerson Therapy." American Cancer Society. http://www.cancer.org/Treatment/TreatmentsandSideEffects/ComplementaryandAlternativeMedicine/DietandNutrition/gerson-therapy (accessed March 22, 2012).

[191] Null, Gary, and Leonard Steinman. "The Politics of Cancer: Part Five." Legacy Tobacco Documents Library. http://legacy.library.ucsf.edu/tid/mtu15b00/pdf?search=%22gary%20null%20cancer%20burton%22 (accessed March 22, 2012).

[192] Ibid.

[193] Ibid.

[194] Pelton, Ross, and Lee Charles Overholser. *Alternatives in Cancer Therapy: The Complete Guide to Non-traditional Treatments*. New York: Simon & Schuster, 1994.

[195] Ibid.

[196] Ibid.

[197] Ibid.

[198] Null, Gary, and Leonard Steinman. "The Politics of Cancer: Part Five." Legacy Tobacco Documents Library. http://legacy.library.ucsf.edu/tid/mtu15b00/pdf?search=%22gary%20null%20cancer%20burton%22 (accessed March 22, 2012).

[199] "Immuno-Technologies, Freeport Bahamas." Cancer Compass An Alternate Route. http://cancercompassalternateroute.com/doctors-and-clinics/immuno-tecnologies-freeport-bahamas/ (accessed November 15, 2013).

[200] Null, Gary. "The Suppression of Cancer Cures." Legacy Tobacco Documents Library. http://legacy.library.ucsf.edu/tid/zsu15b00/pdf?search=%22gary%20null%20cancer%22 (accessed March 20, 2012).

[201] Mercola, Joseph. "Burzynski: The Movie." Mercola.com. http://articles.mercola.com/sites/articles/archive/2011/06/11/burzynski-the-movie.aspx (accessed March 20, 2012).

[202] Ibid.

[203] Ibid.

[204] Ibid.

[205] Elias, Thomas D. "Doctor's Lifesaving Effort Could Land Him in Prison: FDA Ignores Cancer Drug's Success." The Washington Times. http://www.highbeam.com/doc/1G1-56870285.html (accessed March 21, 2012).

[206] Mercola, Joseph. "Burzynski: The Movie." Mercola.com. http://articles.mercola.com/sites/articles/archive/2011/06/11/burzynski-the-movie.aspx (accessed March 20, 2012).

[207] Ibid.

[208] Mercola, Joseph. " Dr. Nicholas Gonzalez on Alternative Cancer Treatments." Mercola. com. http://articles.mercola.com/sites/articles/archive/2011/04/23/dr-nicholas-gonzalez-on-alternative-cancer-treatments.aspx (accessed March 21, 2012).

[209] Aletheia, T.R. *Cancer: An American Conspiracy*. Minneapolis: Mill City Press, 2010.

[210] Lynes, Barry, and John Crane. *The Cancer Cure that Worked! Fifty Years of Suppression*. Toronto, Canada: Marcus Books, 1987.

[211] Lynes, Barry. *The Healing of Cancer: The Cures, the Cover-Ups and the Solution Now*. Queensville, Ontario, Canada: Marcus Books, 1989.

[212] Lynes, Barry, and John Crane. *The Cancer Cure that Worked! Fifty Years of Suppression*. Toronto, Canada: Marcus Books, 1987.

[213] Aletheia, T.R. *Cancer: An American Conspiracy*. Minneapolis: Mill City Press, 2010.

[214] "Complementary Alternative Cancer Therapies—Conventional Cancer Treatment, Chemotherapy—Life Extension Health Concern." Life Extension. http://www.lef.org/protocols/cancer/alternative_cancer_therapies_01.htm (accessed April 1, 2012).

[215] Smallbone, Kieran, David J. Gavaghan, Robert A. Gatenby, and Philip K. Maini. "The Role Of Acidity In Solid Tumour Growth And Invasion." *Journal of Theoretical Biology* 235, no. 4 (2005): 476-484.

[216] Robey, IF, et. al. "Bicarbonate Increases Tumor PH and Inhibits Spontaneous Metastases." Cancer Res 69, no. 6 (2009): 2260-8.

[217] Rofstad, Einar K., et al. "Acidic Extracellular pH Promotes Experimental Metastasis of Human Melanoma Cells in Athymic Nude Mice." *Cancer Research* 66 (2006). http://cancerres.aacrjournals.org/content/66/13/6699.abstract?ijkey=6f1de3dcb24df43416f5003b8f89 2f1b6fd9d741&keytype2=tf_ipsecsha (accessed March 5, 2012).

[218] Cover, CM, et. al. "Indole-3-carbinol Inhibits the Expression of Cyclin-Dependent Kinase-6 and Induces a G1 Cell Cycle Arrest of Human Breast Cancer Cells Independent of Estrogen Receptor Signaling." *J Biol Chem* 273, no. 7 (1998): 3838-47.

[219] Chen, I. et. al. "Indole-3-carbinol and Diindolylmethane As Aryl Hydrocarbon (Ah) Receptor Agonists And Antagonists In T47D Human Breast Cancer Cells." *Biochemical Pharmacology* 51, no. 8 (1996): 1069-1076.

[220] Verhagen, Hans, Henrik E. Poulsen, Steffen Loft, Geert van Poppel, Marianne I. Willems, and Peter J. van Bladeren. "Reduction Of Oxidative DNA-damage In Humans By Brussels Sprouts." *Carcinogenesis* 16, no. 4 (1995): 969-970.

[221] Verhoeven, H. et. al. "Epidemiological Studies on Brassica Vegetables and Cancer Risk." Cancer *Epidemiology, Biomarkers & Prevention* 5, no. 9 (1996): 733-48.

[222] "Discovery May Help Scientists Boost Broccoli's Cancer-Fighting Power." EurekAlert!. http://www.eurekalert.org/pub_releases/2010-10/uoic-dmh102110.php (accessed March 2, 2012).

[223] "Chlorophyll and Chlorophyllin." Linus Pauling Institute at Oregon State University. http://lpi.oregonstate.edu/infocenter/phytochemicals/chlorophylls/index.html#biological_ activity (accessed January 3, 2012).

[224] Cha, Kwang Hyun, Song Yi Koo, and Dong-Un Lee. "Antiproliferative Effects Of Carotenoids Extracted From Chlorella Ellipsoidea And Chlorella Vulgaris On Human Colon Cancer Cells." *Journal of Agricultural and Food Chemistry* 56, no. 22 (2008): 10521-10526.

[225] Mathew, B., R. Sankaranarayanan, P. P. Nair, C. Varghese, T. Somanathan, B. P. Amma.,N. S. Amma, and M. K. Nair. "Evaluation of Chemoprevention of Oral Cancer with Spirulina Fusiformis" *Nutrition and Cancer* 24, no. 2 (1995): 197-202

[226] Maeda, N., et al. "Anti-Cancer Effect of Spinach Glycoglycerolipids as Angiogenesis Inhibitors Based on the Selective Inhibition of DNA Polymerase Activity." *Mini Reviews in*

Medicinal Chemistry 11 (2011). http://www.ncbi.nlm.nih.gov/pubmed/21034405 (accessed March 3, 2012).

227 Blot, William J., You-Hui Zhang, Su-Fang Zheng, Chung S. Yang, Guo-Qing Wang, Sanford Dawsey, Wande Guo, Philip R. Taylor, Jun-Yao Li, Bing Li, Joseph F. Fraumeni, Fusheng Liu, Yu-hai Sun, Joseph Tangrea, Buo-qi Liu, Yu Yu, Guang-Yi Li, and Mitchell Gail. "Nutrition Intervention Trials In Linxian, China: Supplementation With Specific Vitamin/Mineral Combinations, Cancer Incidence, And Disease-Specific Mortality In The General Population." *Journal of the National Cancer Institute* 85, no. 18 (1993): 1483-1491.

228 Tanaka, T., M.Shminimizu, and H.Moriwaki. "Cancer Chemoprevention by Carotenoids." *Molecules* 14;17, no. 3 (2012): 3202-42. http://www.ncbi.nlm.nih.gov/pubmed/22418926 (accessed March 27, 2012).

229 Pinela, J. et al. "Nutritional Composition and Antioxidant Activity of Four Tomato (Lycopersiconesculentum L.) Farmer' Varieties in Northeastern Portugal Home Gardens." *Food and Chemical Toxicology* 50, no. (3-4) (2011): 829-34.

230 "Fiber." University of Maryland Medical Center. http://www.umm.edu/altmed/articles/fiber-000303.htm (accessed December 3, 2012).

231 "High-Fiber Diet May Thwart Colon Cancer." HealthDay, USATODAY.com. http://usa-today30.usatoday.com/news/health/medical/health/medical/cancer/story/2011-11-11/High-fiber-diet-may-help-thwart-colon-cancer/51168932/1 (accessed March 28, 2012).

232 "Uterine Cancer—2—Endometrial Cancer, Vitamin A, Vitamin C—Life Extension Health Concern." Life Extension. http://www.lef.org/protocols/cancer/uterine_cancer_02.htm (accessed March 28, 2012).

233 Owen, R W, R Haubner, G Wertele, W E Hull, B Spiegelhalder, and H Bartsch. "Olives And Olive Oil In Cancer Prevention." *European Journal of Cancer Prevention* 13, no. 4 (2004): 319-326.

234 Menendez, JA, and R Lupu. "Mediterranean Dietary Traditions for the Molecular Treatment of Human Cancer: Anti-oncogenic actions of the main olive oil's monounsaturated fatty acid oleic acid." *Curr Pharm Biotechnol* 7, no. 6 (2006): 495-502.

235 Menendez, Javier A, Alejandro Vazquez-Martin, Rocio Garcia-Villalba, Alegria Carrasco-Pancorbo, Cristina Oliveras-Ferraros, Alberto Fernandez-Gutierrez, and Antonio Segura-Carretero. "Anti-HER2 (erbB-2) Oncogene Effects Of Phenolic Compounds Directly Isolated From Commercial Extra-Virgin Olive Oil (EVOO)." *BMC Cancer* 8, no. 1 (2008): 377.

236 Choi, Hyun, Do Lim, and Jung Park. "Induction Of G1 And G2/M Cell Cycle Arrests By The Dietary Compound 3,3'-diindolylmethane In HT-29 Human Colon Cancer Cells." *BMC Gastroenterology* 9, no. 1 (2009): 39.

237 Bhatnagar, N., X. Li, Y. Chen, X. Zhou, S. H. Garrett, and B. Guo. "3,3'-Diindolylmethane Enhances The Efficacy Of Butyrate In Colon Cancer Prevention Through Down-Regulation Of Survivin." *Cancer prevention research* 2, no. 6 (2009): 581-589.

238 Schnäbele, K., et al. "Effects of Carrot and Tomato Juice Consumption on FaecalMarkers Relevant to Colon Carcinogenesis in Humans." *The British Journal of Nutrition* 99, no. 3 (2008): 606-613. http://www.ncbi.nlm.nih.gov/pubmed/18254985 (accessed March 13, 2012).

239 "Tea." Linus Pauling Institute at Oregon State University. http://lpi.oregonstate.edu/info-center/phytochemicals/tea (accessed January 3, 2012).

240 "Green Tea Extract Appears to Keep Cancer in Check in Majority of CLL Patients." Mayo Clinic. http://www.mayoclinic.org/news2010-rst/5833.html (accessed January 3, 2012).

241 Okello, EJ, GJ McDougall, S Kumar, and CJ Seal. "In Vitro Protective Effects of Colon-Available Extract of Camellia Sinensis (tea) Against Hydrogen Peroxide and Beta-amyloid (Aβ((1-42))) Induced Cytotoxicity in Differentiated PC12 Cells.." *Phytomedicine* 15, no. 18 (2011): 691-6.

242 Israilides, C., D. Kletsas, D. Arapoglou, A. Philippoussis, H. Pratsinis, A. Ebringerová, V. Hříbalová, and S.E. Harding. "In Vitro Cytostatic And Immunomodulatory Properties Of The Medicinal Mushroom Lentinula Edodes."Phytomedicine 15, no. 6-7 (2008): 512-519.

243 Chan, J. Y., et al. "Enhancement of In Vitro and In Vivo Anticancer Activities of Polysaccharide Peptide from Grifolafrondosa by Chemical Modifications." *Pharmaceutical Biology* 49, no. 11 (2011): 1114-1120

244 Masuda, Y. "A Polysaccharide Extracted from GrifolafrondosaEnhances the Anti-tumor Activity of Bone Marrow-Derived Dendritic Cell-Based Immunotherapy against Murine Colon Cancer." *Cancer Immunology, Immunotherapy* 59, no. 10 (2009): 1531-41.

245 Fullerton, S. A. "Induction of Apoptosis in Human Prostatic Cancer Cells with Beta-glucan (MaitakeMushroom Polysaccharide)." *Molecular Urology* 4, no. 1 (2000): 7-13.

246 Tanaka, K., et al. "Oral Ingestion of LentinulaedodesMycelia Extract Inhibits B16 Melanoma Growth via Mitigation of Regulatory T Cell-Mediated Immunosuppression." *Cancer Science* 102, no. 3 (2011): 516-21.

247 Israilides, C., et al. "In Vitro Cytostatic and Immunomodulatory Properties of the Medicinal Mushrooms LentinulaEdodes." *Phytomedicine,* June 2008.

248 Sliva, Daniel. "Ganoderma Lucidum (Reishi) in Cancer Treatment." *Integrative Cancer Therapies* 2, no. 4 (2003): 358-364.

249 Das, Shonkor Kumar, Mina Masuda, Akihiko Sakurai, and Mikio Sakakibara. "Medicinal Uses Of The Mushroom Cordyceps Militaris: Current State And Prospects." *Fitoterapia* 81, no. 8 (2010): 961-968.

250 Chen, S., L. S. Adams, M. Belury, G. E. Shrode, S. L. Kwok, J. J. Ye, G. Hur, S. Phung, S.-R. Oh, and D. Williams. "Anti-Aromatase Activity Of Phytochemicals In White Button Mushrooms (Agaricus Bisporus)." *CANCER RESEARCH* 66, no. 24 (2006): 12026-12034.

251 Burtin, Patricia. "Nutritional Value of Seaweed." *Electronic Journal of Environmental and Food Chemistry* 2 (2003). http://www.scribd.com/doc/93899794/Nutritional-Seawaed (accessed January 3, 2012).

252 Ermakova, S, R Sokolova, SM Kim, BH Um, V Isakov, and T Zvyagintseva. "Fucoidans From Brown Seaweeds Sargassum Hornery, Eclonia Cava, Costaria Costata: Structural characteristics and anticancer activity." *Appl Biochem Biotechnol* 164, no. 6 (2011): 841-50.

253 Gali-Muhtasib, H., M. Diab-Assaf, C. Boltze, J. Al-Hmaira, R. Hartig, etal. "Thymoquinone Extracted from Black Seed Triggers Apoptotic Cell Death in Human Colorectal Cancer Cells Via a p53-dependent Mechanism." *Internatinal Journal of Oncology* 25, no. 2 (2004):857-66.

254 Salim, Elsayed I., and Shoji Fukushima. "Chemopreventive Potential Of Volatile Oil From Black Cumin (Nigella Sativa L.) Seeds Against Rat Colon Carcinogenesis." *Nutrition and Cancer 45*, no. 2 (2003): 195-202.

255 S. Duessel, et al. "Growth Inhibition of Human Colon Cancer Cells by Plant Compounds." *Clinical Laboratory Science* 21, no. 3 (2008): 151-7.

256 Chan, M. "Effects Of Three Dietary Phytochemicals From Tea, Rosemary And Turmeric On Inflammation-induced Nitrite Production." *Cancer Letters* 96, no. 1 (1995): 23-29.

257 S. Cheung, et al. "Anti-proliferative and Antioxidant Properties of Rosemary RosmarinusOfficinalis." *Oncology Reports* 17, no. 6 (2007): 1525-31.

258 Ho, C.-T., T. Ferraro, Q. Chen, R. T. Rosen, and M.-T. Huang. "ChemInform Abstract: Phytochemicals In Teas And Rosemary And Their Cancer-Preventive Properties." *ChemInform* 25, no. 15 (1994): 2-19.

259 "Pepper Component Hot Enough to Trigger Suicide in Prostate Cancer Cells." Cedars-Sinai Hospital. http://www.eurekalert.org/pub_releases/2006-03/aafc-pch031306.php (accessed 15 Mar, 2006.)

260 Johnson, J. J. "Carnosol: APromising Anti-cancer and Anti-inflammatory Agent." *Cancer Letters* 305, no. 1 (2011): 1-7. http://www.ncbi.nlm.nih.gov/pubmed/21382660 (accessed March 12, 2012).

261 "Parsley, Celery Carry Crucial Component for Fight against Breast Cancer, Study Suggests." Science Daily. http://www.sciencedaily.com/releases/2011/05/110509122732.htm (accessed March 21, 2012).

262 Roberts II, L. Jackson, Maret G. Traber, and Balz Frei. "Vitamins E And C In The Prevention Of Cardiovascular Disease And Cancer In Men." Free Radical Biology and Medicine 46, no. 11 (2009): 1558-1558.

263 Zhang, S. et. al. "Dietary Carotenoids and Vitamins A, C, and E and Risk of Breast Cancer." *J Natl Cancer Inst* 17, no. 91 (1999): 547-56.

264 Feliz, HR, and S Mobarhan. "Does Vitamin C Intake Slow the Progression of Gastric Cancer in Helicobacter Pylori-Infected Populations?." *Nutr* Rev 60, no. 1 (2002): 34-6.

265 Chen, Q., M. G. Espey, A. Y. Sun, C. Pooput, K. L. Kirk, M. C. Krishna, D. B. Khosh, J. Drisko, and M. Levine. "From The Cover: Pharmacologic Doses Of Ascorbate Act As A Prooxidant And Decrease Growth Of Aggressive Tumor Xenografts In Mice." *Proceedings of the National Academy of Sciences* 105, no. 32 (2008): 11105-11109.

266 Drisko, JA, J Chapman, and VJ Hunter. "The Use of Antioxidants with First-Line Chemotherapy in Two Cases of Ovarian Cancer." *J Am Coll Nutr* 22, no. 2 (2003): 118-23.

267 Gonzalez, M. J.. "Orthomolecular Oncology Review: Ascorbic Acid And Cancer 25 Years Later." *Integrative Cancer Therapies* 4, no. 1 (2005): 32-44.

268 Moss, R. W.. "Should Patients Undergoing Chemotherapy And Radiotherapy Be Prescribed Antioxidants?." *Integrative Cancer Therapies* 5, no. 1 (2006): 63-82.

269 van de Mark, K, et al. "Alpha-lipoic Acid Induces p27 Kip-Dependent Cell Cycle Arrest in Non-transformed Cell Lines and Apoptosis in Tumor Cell Lines." *Journal of Cellular Physiology* 194, no. 3 (2003): 325-40.

270 Lee, H. S., et al.; "Alpha-Lipoic Acid Reduces Matrix Metalloproteinase Activity in MDA-MB-231 Human Breast Cancer Cells." *Nutrition Research* 30, no. 6 (2010): 403-9.

271 Myzak, M. C., and A. C. Carr. "Myeloperoxidase-Dependent Caspase-3 Activation and Apoptosis in HL-60 Cells: Protection by the Antioxidants Ascorbate and (Dihydro)lipoic-Acid." *Redox Report* 7, no. 1 (2002): 47-53. http://www.ncbi.nlm.nih.gov/pubmed/11981455 (accessed March 13, 2012).

272 Brown, M. D. "Promotion of Prostatic Metastatic Migration towards Human Bone Marrow Stoma by Omega 6 and Its Inhibition by Omega 3 PUFAs." *British Journal of Cancer* 94, no. 6 (2006): 842-53.

273 Gago-Dominguez, M. "Opposing Effects of Dietary n-3 and n-6 Fatty Acids on Mammary Carcinogenesis: The Singapore Chinese Health Study." *British Journal of Cancer* 89, no. 9 (2003): 1686-92.

274 MacLean, C., et al. "Effects of Omega-3 Fatty Acids on Cancer." *AHRQ Evidence Reports*, February 2005.

275 Prakash, Pankaj, Norman I. Krinsky, and Robert M. Russell. "Retinoids, Carotenoids, And Human Breast Cancer Cell Cultures: A Review Of Differential Effects." *Nutrition Reviews* 58, no. 6 (2000): 170-176.

276 "Vitamin A May Slash Melanoma Risk, Especially in Women." LiveScience. http://www.livescience.com/18755-melanoma-risk-vitamin-women.html (accessed March 28, 2012).

277 de Klerk, NH. Et. al. "Vitamin A and Cancer Prevention II: comparison of the effects of retinol and beta-carotene." *Int J Cancer* 75, no. 3 (1998): 362-7.

[278] Sivakumaran, Muttuswamy. "Role of Vitamin A Deficiency in the Pathogenesis of MyeloproliferativeDisorders." *Blood Journal.* http://bloodjournal.hematologylibrary.org/content/98/5/1636.full (accessed March 28, 2012).

[279] Li, K., et al. "The Effect of Vitamin A Deficiency in Maternal Rats on Tumor Formation in Filial Rats." *Journal of Pediatric Surgery* 44, no. 3 (2009): 565-570. http://www.ncbi.nlm.nih.gov/pubmed/19302860 (accessed March 12, 2012).

[280] Ruano-Ravina, A, A Figueiras, and JM Barros-Dios. "Diet and Lung Cancer: A new approach." *Eur J Cancer Prev* 9, no. 6 (2000): 395-400.

[281] DiGiovanna, John J. "Retinoid Chemoprevention In Patients At High Risk For Skin Cancer." *Medical and Pediatric Oncology* 36, no. 5 (2001): 564-567.

[282] Null, Gary. *The Complete Encyclopedia of Natural Healing.* New York: Kensington, 1998.

[283] E. Cho et al. "Premenopausal Intakes of Vitamins A, C, and E, Folate, and Carotenoids, and Risk of Breast Cancer." *Cancer Epidemiology, Biomarkers and Prevention* 12, no. 8 (2003): 713-20.

[284] Zhang, Shumin, et al. "Dietary Carotenoids and Vitamins A, C, and E and Risk of Breast Cancer." *Journal of the National Cancer Institute* 91, no. 6 (1999): 547-56.

[285] Knekt, Paul."Dietary Flavonoids and the Risk of Lung Cancer and Other Malignant Neoplasms." *American Journal of Epidemiology* 146, no. 3 (1997):223-230.

[286] Le Marchand, Loïc, et al. "Intake of Flavonoids and Lung Cancer." *Journal of the National Cancer Institute* 92, no. 2 (1999): 154-60.

[287] Cui, Yan, Qing-Yi Lu, Thomas M. Mack, Wendy Cozen, Lin Cai, Jenny T. Mao, Donald P. Tashkin, Sander Greenland, Hal Morgenstern, and Zuo-Feng Zhang. "Dietary Flavonoid Intake And Lung Cancer—A Population-based Case-control Study." *Cancer* 112, no. 10 (2008): 2241-2248.

[288] "Vitamin E." Linus Pauling Institute at Oregon State University. http://lpi.oregonstate.edu/infocenter/vitamins/vitaminE/ (accessed March 21, 2012).

[289] "Vitamin E in Front Line of Prostate Cancer Fight." Science Daily. http://www.sciencedaily.com/releases/2010/10/101019111718.htm (accessed March 8, 2012).

[290] Null, Gary. *The Complete Encyclopedia of Natural Healing.* New York: Kensington, 1998.

[291] Li, Lu, Zhiling Qi, Jin Qian, Fuyong Bi, Jun Lv, Lei Xu, Ling Zhang, Hongyu Chen, and Renbing Jia. "Induction Of Apoptosis In Hepatocellular Carcinoma Smmc-7721 Cells By Vitamin K2 Is Associated With P53 And Independent Of The Intrinsic Apoptotic Pathway." *Molecular and Cellular Biochemistry* 342, no. 1-2 (2010): 125-131.

[292] Nimptsch, Katharina. "Dietary Vitamin K Intake in Relation to Cancer Incidence and Mortality: Results from the Heidelberg Cohort of the European Prospective Investigation into Cancer and Nutrition." *American Journal of Clinical Nutrition* 10.3945 (2010). http://www.ajcn.org/content/early/2010/03/24/ajcn.2009.28691.abstract (accessed March 13, 2012).

[293] Kaneda, Makoto, Dan Zhang, Rajib Bhattacharjee, Ken-ichi Nakahama, Shigeki Arii, and Ikuo Morita. "Vitamin K2 Suppresses Malignancy Of HuH7 Hepatoma Cells Via Inhibition Of Connexin 43." *Cancer Letters* 263, no. 1 (2008): 53-60.

[294] Amaral, A. F. S., K. P. Cantor, D. T. Silverman, and N. Malats. "Selenium And Bladder Cancer Risk: A Meta-analysis." *Cancer Epidemiology Biomarkers & Prevention* 19, no. 9 (2010): 2407-2415.

[295] Duffield-Lillico, A. J., et al. "Selenium Supplementation, Baseline Plasma Selenium Status and Incidence of Prostate Cancer: An Analysis of the Complete Treatment Period of the Nutritional Prevention of Cancer Trial." *BJU International* 91, no. 7 (2003): 608-12.

[296] Bleys, J., et al. "Serum Selenium Levels and All-Cause, Cancer, and Cardiovascular Mortality among U.S. Adults." *Archives of Internal Medicine* 168, no. 4 (2008): 404-10.

[297] Syed, D. N., N. Khan, F. Afaq, and H. Mukhtar. "Chemoprevention Of Prostate Cancer Through Dietary Agents: Progress And Promise." *Cancer Epidemiology Biomarkers & Prevention* 16, no. 11 (2007): 2193-2203.

[298] Lah, JJ, W Cui, and KQ Hu. "Effects and Mechanisms of Silibinin on Human Hepatoma Cell Lines." *World J Gastroenterol* 13, no. 40 (2007): 5299-305.

[299] Kiefer, Dale. "Report: A New Weapon to Fight Prostate Cancer." *Life Extension Magazine*, November 2005. http://www.lef.org/magazine/mag2005/nov2005_report_prostate_01.htm (accessed March 3, 2012).

[300] Null, Gary. *The Complete Encyclopedia of Natural Healing*. New York: Kensington, 1998.

[301] Sakano, K., et al. "Suppression of Azoxymethane-Induced Colonic Premalignant Lesion Formation by Coenzyme Q10 in Rats." *Asian Pacific Journal of Cancer Prevention* 7, no. 4 (2006): 599-603.

[302] Rusciani, L., et al. "Recombinant Interferon Alpha-2b and Coenzyme Q10 as a Postsurgical Adjuvant Therapy for Melanoma: A 3-Year Trial with Recombinant Interferon-Alpha and 5-Year Follow-Up." *Melanoma Research* 17, no. 3 (2007): 177-83.

[303] Folkers, Karl, Anders Osterborg, Magnus Nylander, Manabu Morita, and Haken Mellstedt. "Activities Of Vitamin Q10in Animal Models And A Serious Deficiency In Patients With Cancer." *Biochemical and Biophysical Research Communications* 234, no. 2 (1997): 296-299.

[304] Kaur, M., C. Agarwal, and R. Agarwal. "Anticancer And Cancer Chemopreventive Potential Of Grape Seed Extract And Other Grape-Based Products." *Journal of Nutrition* 139, no. 9 (2009): 1806S-1812S.

[305] Radhakrishnan, S. "Resveratrol Potentiates Grape Seed Extract Induced Human Colon Cancer Cell Apoptosis." *Frontiers in Bioscience* 1, no. 3 (2011): 1509-23.

[306] Raina, K., R. P. Singh, R. Agarwal, and C. Agarwal. "Oral Grape Seed Extract Inhibits Prostate Tumor Growth And Progression In TRAMP Mice." *CANCER RESEARCH* 67, no. 12 (2007): 5976-5982.

[307] Chen,Changjie, et al. "Grape Seed Extract InhibitsProliferation of Breast Cancer Cell MCF-7 and Decrease the Gene Expression of Survivin; China Journal of Chinese MateriaMedica 34, no. 4 (2009): 433-7.

[308] Null, Gary. *The Complete Encyclopedia of Natural Healing*. New York: Kensington, 1998.

[309] Wise, D., and C. Thompson." Glutamine Addiction: A New Therapeutic Target in Cancer." *Trends in Biochemical Sciences* 35, no. 8 (2010): 427-33

[310] Villareal, DT, and JO Holloszy. "Effect of DHEA on Abdominal Fat and Insulin Action in Elderly Women and Men: a randomized controlled trial.." *JAMA* 292, no. 10 (2004): 2243-8.

[311] Smith, Timothy J. *Renewal: The Anti-Aging Revolution*. Rodale Press, 1998.

[312] Jung, B., and N. Ahmad. "Melatonin In Cancer Management: Progress And Promise." *CANCER RESEARCH* 66, no. 20 (2006): 9789-9793.

[313] Megdal, S, C Kroenke, F Laden, E Pukkala, and E Schernhammer. "Night Work And Breast Cancer Risk: A Systematic Review And Meta-analysis." *European Journal of Cancer* 41, no. 13 (2005): 2023-2032.

[314] Lissoni, Paolo, Sandro Barni, Antonio Ardizzoia, Gabriele Tancini, Ario Conti, and George Maestroni. "A Randomized Study With The Pineal Hormone Melatonin Versus Supportive Care Alone In Patients With Brain Metastases Due To Solid Neoplasms." *Cancer* 73, no. 3 (1994): 699-701.

[315] Schernhammer, E. S., and S. E. Hankinson. "Urinary Melatonin Levels And Postmenopausal Breast Cancer Risk In The Nurses' Health Study Cohort." *Cancer Epidemiology Biomarkers & Prevention* 18, no. 1 (2009): 74-79.

[316] Park, S.Y., et al. "Melatonin Suppresses Tumor Angiogenesis by Inhibiting HIF-1alpha Stabilization Under Hypoxia." *Journal of Pineal Research* 48, no. 2 (2010): 178-84.

[317] Beuth, J.. "Proteolytic Enzyme Therapy In Evidence-Based Complementary Oncology: Fact Or Fiction?." *Integrative Cancer Therapies* 7, no. 4 (2008): 311-316.

[318] Yamashita, Keishi, et al. "A Tumor-Suppressive Role for Trypsin in Human Cancer Progression." *Cancer Research* 63 (2003). http://cancerres.aacrjournals.org/content/63/20/6575.full (accessed March 5, 2012).

[319] Wald, M., et al. "Mixture of Trypsin, Chymotrypsin and Papain Reduces Formation of Metasteses and Extends Survival Time of C57B16 Mice with Syngeneic Melanoma B16." *Cancer Chemotherapy and Pharmacology* 47, (2001): S16-22.

[320] R, Báez, et al. . "In vivo antitumoral activity of stem pineapple (Ananas comosus) bromelain.." *Planta Medica* 73, no. 13 (2007): 1377-83. http://www.ncbi.nlm.nih.gov/pubmed/17893836 (accessed January 2, 2013).

[321] Larsson, S.C., et al. "High-Fat Dairy Food and Conjugated Linoleic Acid Intakes in Relation to Colorectal Cancer." *American Journal of Clinical Nutrition*, 2005. vol. 82 no. 4 894-900

[322] Chen, B. Q., et al. "Inhibitory Effects of c9, t11-Conjugated Linoleic Acid." *The World Journal of Gastroenterology* 9, no. 9 (2003): 1909-14.

[323] Aro, Antti, Satu Männistö, Irma Salminen, Marja-Leena Ovaskainen, Vesa Kataja, and Matti Uusitupa. "Inverse Association Between Dietary And Serum Conjugated Linoleic Acid And Risk Of Breast Cancer In Postmenopausal Women." *Nutrition and Cancer* 38, no. 2 (2000): 151-157.

[324] Lp, Clement, Joseph A. Scimeca, and Henry J. Thompson. "Conjugated Linoleic Acid. A Powerful Anticarcinogen From Animal Fat Sources." *Cancer* 74, no. S3 (1994): 1050-1054.

[325] Kritchevsky, D. "Antimutagenic and Some Other Effects of Conjugated Linoleic Acid." *Br J Nutr* 83, no. 5 (2000): 459-65.

[326] Bhattacharya, A, J Banu, M Rahman, J Causey, and G Fernandes. "Biological Effects Of Conjugated Linoleic Acids In Health And Disease." *The Journal of Nutritional Biochemistry* 17, no. 12 (2006): 789-810.

[327] Johnson, Kim D., Avraham Raz, Olga V. Glinskii, Vladislav V. Glinsky, Kenneth J. Pienta, Gennadi V. Glinsky, Virginia H. Huxley, Carolyn J. Henry, Douglas C. Anthony, Thomas P. Mawhinney, James R. Turk, and Valeri V. Mossine. "Galectin-3 As A Potential Therapeutic Target In Tumors Arising From Malignant Endothelia." *Neoplasia* 9, no. 8 (2007): 662-670.

[328] Gupta, Gaorav P., and Joan Massagué. "Cancer Metastasis: Building A Framework." *Cell* 127, no. 4 (2006): 679-695.

[329] Strum, S., M. Scholz, J. McDermed, M. McCulloch, I. Eliaz. "Modified Citrus Pectin Slows PSA Doubling Time: A Pilot Clinical Trial." Paper presented at the International Conference on Diet and Prevention of Cancer, May 1999, Tampere, Finland.

[330] Guess, B W, M C Scholz, S B Strum, R Y Lam, H J Johnson, and R I Jennrich. "Modified Citrus Pectin (MCP) Increases The Prostate-specific Antigen Doubling Time In Men With Prostate Cancer: A Phase II Pilot Study." *Prostate Cancer and Prostatic Diseases* 6, no. 4 (2003): 301-304.

[331] Ushida, Y. et. al. "Inhibitory Effects of Bovine Lactoferrin on Intestinal Polyposis in the Apc(Min) Mouse." *Cancer Lett* 134, no. 2 (1998): 141-5.

[332] Yoo, Yung-Choon, Shikiko Watanabe, Ryosuke Watanabe, Katsusuke Hata, Kei-ichi Shimazaki, and Ichiro Azuma. "Bovine Lactoferrin And Lactoferricin, A Peptide Derived From Bovine Lactoferrin, Inhibit Tumor Metastasis In Mice." *Cancer Science* 88, no. 2 (1997): 184-190.

[333] Sakamoto, N. "Antitumor Effect of Human Lactoferrin Against Newly Established Human Pancreatic Cancer Cell Line SPA." *Gan To Kagaku Ryoho 25, no.* 10 (1998): 1557-63.

[334] Tsuda, H. et. al. "Inhibition of Azoxymethane Initiated Colon Tumor and Aberrant Crypt Foci Development by Bovine Lactoferrin Administration in F344 Rats." *Adv Exp Med Biol* 443 (1998): 273-84.

[335] Li, Jian, Huai-Jun Tu, Jie Li, Ge Dai, Yu-Cheng Dai, Qiong Wu, Qing-Zhi Shi, Qing Cao, and Zhen-Jiang Li. "N-acetyl Cysteine Inhibits Human Signet Ring Cell Gastric Cancer Cell Line (SJ-89) Cell Growth By Inducing Apoptosis And DNA Synthesis Arrest." *European Journal of Gastroenterology & Hepatology* 19, no. 9 (2007): 769-774.

[336] Yanh, J, Y Su, and A Richmond. "Antioxidants tiron and N-acetyl-L-cysteine differentially mediate apoptosis in melanoma cells via a reactive oxygen species-independent NF-kappaB pathway." *Free Radic Biol Med* 42, no. 9 (2007): 1369-80.

[337] Balansky, Roumen, Gancho Ganchev, Marietta Iltcheva, Vernon E. Steele, and Silvio De Flora. "Prevention Of Cigarette Smoke-induced Lung Tumors In Mice By Budesonide, Phenethyl Isothiocyanate, And-acetylcysteine." *International Journal of Cancer* 126, no. 5 (2009): 1047-54

[338] Guan, D, Y Xu, M Yang, H Wang, and Z Shen. "N-acetyl Cysteine and Penicillamine Induce Apoptosis via the ER Stress Response-Signaling Pathway." *Mol Carcinog* 49, no. 1 (2010): 68-74.

[339] Fares, R., et al. "The Antioxidant and Anti-proliferative Activity of the Lebanese OleaEuropaeaExtract." *Plant Foods in Human Nutrition* 66, no. 1 (2011): 58-63.

[340] Bouallagui, Zouhaier, Junkuy Han, Hiroko Isoda, and Sami Sayadi. "Hydroxytyrosol Rich Extract From Olive Leaves Modulates Cell Cycle Progression In MCF-7 Human Breast Cancer Cells." *Food and Chemical Toxicology* 49, no. 1 (2011): 179-184.

[341] Mijatovic, Sanja A., Gordana S. Timotijevic, Djordje M. Miljkovic, Julijana M. Radovic, Danijela D. Maksimovic-Ivanic, Dragana P. Dekanski, and Stanislava D. Stosic-Grujicic. "Multiple Antimelanoma Potential Of Dry Olive Leaf Extract." *International Journal of Cancer* 128, no. 8 (2011): 1955-1965.

[342] Arthur, G, and R Bittman. "The Inhibition of Cell Signaling Pathways by Antitumor Ether Lipids." *Biochim Biophys Acta* 1390, no. 1 (1998): 85-102.

[343] Samadder, P, C Richards, R Bittman, RP Bhullar, and G Arthur. "The Antitumor Ether Lipid 1-Q-octadecyl-2-O-methyl-rac-glycerophosphocholine (ET-18-OCH3) Inhibits the Association Between Ras and Raf-1." *Anticancer Res* 23, no. 3B (2003): 2291-5.

[344] Pédrono, Frédérique, Naïm A Khan, and Alain B Legrand. "Regulation Of Calcium Signalling By 1-O-alkylglycerols In Human Jurkat T Lymphocytes." *Life Sciences* 74, no. 22 (2004): 2793-2801.

[345] Brohult, A, and J Holmberg. "Alkoxyglycerols in the Treatment of Leukopaenia Caused y Irradiation."*Nature* 174, no. 4441 (1954): 1102-3.

[346] Jang, M. et. al. "Cancer Chemopreventive Activity of Resveratrol, a Natural Product Derived from Grapes." *Science* 275, no. 5297 (1997): 218-20.

[347] Fulda, S, and K Debatin. "Resveratrol Modulation Of Signal Transduction In Apoptosis And Cell Survival: A Mini-review." *Cancer Detection and Prevention* 30, no. 3 (2006): 217-223.

[348] Woo, JH. Et. al. "Resveratrol Inhibits Phorbol Myristate Acetate-Induced Matrix Metalloproteinase-9 Expression by Inhibiting JNK and PKC Delta Signal Transduction." *Oncogene* 23, no. 10 (2004): 1845-53.

[349] Ciolino, HP, and GC Yeh. "Inhibition of Aryl Hydrocarbon-Induced Cytochrome P-450 1A1 Enzyme Activity and CYP1A1 Expression by Resveratrol." *Mol Pharmacol* 56, no. 4 (1999): 760-7.

[350] Joe, AK. et. al. "Resveratrol Induces Growth Inhibition, S-phase Arrest, Apoptosis, and Changes in Biomarker Expression in Several Human Cancer Cell Lines." *Clin Cancer Res* 8, no. 3 (2002): 893-903.

[351] "Cancer Research—Bindweed." The Riordan Clinic Health Center in Wichita, KS. http://www.riordanclinic.org/research/research-studies/cancer/bindweed/ (accessed March 21, 2012).

[352] Riordan, N. H., X. Meng, and H. D. Riordan. "Effects of Cell Wall Extracts of Gram Positive Bacteria (MPGC) on Human Immunity and Tumor Growth in Animals." Presentation at Comprehensive Cancer Care 2000, Arlington, Virginia, June 2000.

[353] Prasad, A.S., et al. "Dietary Zinc and Prostate Cancer in the TRAMP Mouse Model." *Journal of Medicinal Food* 13, no. 1 (2010): 70-6.

[354] Epstein, M. M., K. Fall, J.-E. Johansson, S.-O. Andersson, N. Hakansson, A. Wolk, E. L. Giovannucci, O. Andren, J. L. Kasperzyk, and L. A. Mucci. "Dietary Zinc And Prostate Cancer Survival In A Swedish Cohort." *American Journal of Clinical Nutrition* 93, no. 3 (2011): 586-593.

[355] Song, Won O., Ock Kyoung Chun, Inkyeong Hwang, Han Seung Shin, Bong-Gwan Kim, Kun Soo Kim, Sang-Yun Lee, Dayeon Shin, and Sung G. Lee. "Soy Isoflavones As Safe Functional Ingredients." *Journal of Medicinal Food* 10, no. 4 (2007): 571-580.

[356] "Soy Compound May Halt Spread of Prostate Cancer." Science Daily. http://www.science-daily.com/releases/2008/03/080314085038.htm (accessed March 29, 2012).

[357] Aboutalebi, S., et al. "Immune Protection, Natural Products, and Skin Cancer: Is There Anything New under the Sun?" *Journal of Drugs in Dermatology* 5, no. 6 (2006): 512-7

[358] Pecere, Teresa, et al. "Aloe-emodin Is a New Type of Anticancer Agent with Selective Activity against Neuroectodermal Tumors." *Cancer Research* 60 (2000). http://cancerres.aacrjournals.org/content/60/11/2800.short (accessed March 14, 2012).

[359] Corsi, M. M., et al. "The Therapeutic Potential of Aloe Vera in Tumor-Bearing Rats." *International Journal of Tissue Reactions* 20, no. 4 (1998): 115-118. http://ukpmc.ac.uk/abstract/MED/10093794/reload=0;jsessionid=tdlDotXQVWctw7ukpVz9.2 (accessed March 12, 2012).

[360] Duan, P. and Z. Wang. "Clinical Study on Effect of Astragalus in Efficacy Enhancing and Toxicity Reducing of Chemotherapy in Patients of Malignant Tumor." *Zhongguo Zhong Xi Yi Jie He Za Zhi* 22, no. 7 (2002): 515-7

[361] Cui, Rutao, Jinchun He, Baoen Wang, Fukui Zhang, Guangyong Chen, Shanshan Yin, and Hong Shen. "Suppressive Effect Of Astragalus Membranaceus Bunge On Chemical Hepatocarcinogenesis In Rats." *Cancer Chemotherapy and Pharmacology* 51, no. 1 (2003): 75-80.

[362] Cho, W, and K Leung. "In Vitro And In Vivo Anti-tumor Effects Of Astragalus Membranaceus." *Cancer Letters* 252, no. 1 (2007): 43-54.

[363] Auyeung, K.k., P.k. Woo, P.c. Law, and J.k. Ko. "Astragalus Saponins Modulate Cell Invasiveness And Angiogenesis In Human Gastric Adenocarcinoma Cells." *Journal of Ethnopharmacology* 141, no. 2 (2011): 635-41.

[364] Pretner, E. et. al. "Cancer-Related Overexpression of the Peripheral-Type Benzodiazepine Receptor and Cytostatic Anticancer Effects of Ginkgo Biloba Extract (EGb 761)." *Anticancer Res* 26, no. 1A (2006): 9-22.

[365] Xu, AH. et. al. "Therapeutic Mechanism of Ginkgo Biloba Exocarp Polysaccharides on Gastric Cancer." *World J Gastroenterol* 9, no. 11 (2003): 2424-7.

[366] Ye, B, M Aponte, Y Dai, L Li, M Ho, A Vitonis, D Edwards, T Huang, and D Cramer. "Ginkgo Biloba And Ovarian Cancer Prevention: Epidemiological And Biological Evidence." *Cancer Letters* 251, no. 1 (2007): 43-52.

[367] Block, Keith, and Mark Mead. "Immune System Effects of Echinacea, Ginseng, and Astragalus: A Review." *Integrative Cancer Therapies* 3 (2003). http://www.comilac.com.tr/uploads/pdf/galuskaynak2.pdf (accessed March 6, 2012).

[368] Fleischauer, A. et al. "Garlic Consumption and Cancer Prevention: Meta-analyses of Colorectal and Stomach Cancers." *American Journal of Clinical Nutrition* 72, no. 4 (2000): 1047-52.

[369] Nqo, S. et al. "Does Garlic Reduce Risk of Colorectal Cancer? A Systematic Review." *Journal of Nutrition* 137, no. 10 (2007): 2264-9.

[370] Hong, Y.S., et al. "Effects of Allyl Sulfur Compounds and Garlic Extract on the Expression of Bcl-2, Bax, and p53 in Non Small Cell Lung Cancer Cell Lines." *Experimental and Molecular Medicine* 32, no. 3 (2000):127-34.

[371] Bhatia, Kanchan, et al. "Protective Effect of S-allylcysteine against Cyclophosphamide-Induced Bladder Hemorrhagic Cystitis in Mice." *Food and Chemical Toxicology* 46, no. 11 (2008). http://www.sciencedirect.com/science/article/pii/S0278691508004274 (accessed March 8, 2012).

[372] "Dietary Ginger May Work Against Cancer Growth." Science Daily. http://www.science-daily.com/releases/2003/10/031029064357.htm (accessed March 29, 2012).

[373] Jeong, C.-H., H. Jiang, H. Li, Y.-J. Jeon, J.-H. Shim, H.-G. Kim, Y.-Y. Cho, A. Pugliese, A. M. Bode, and Z. Dong. "[6]-Gingerol Suppresses Colon Cancer Growth By Targeting Leukotriene A4 Hydrolase." *CANCER RESEARCH* 69, no. 13 (2009): 5584-5591.

[374] Liu, R.et. al. "Expression and Function of Intracellular Fatty Acid-Binding Proteins in Human Malignant Glioma Cells and Tissues." Presentation at the 97th Annual Meeting of the American Association for Cancer Research. Washington, D.C., 2006.

[375] Borger, J. Everett. "How Curcumin Protects against Cancer." *Life Extension Magazine.* http://www.lef.org/magazine/mag2011/mar2011_How-Curcumin-Protects-Against-Cancer_01.htm?source=search&key=curcumin percent20cancer (accessed March 9, 2012).

[376] Ravindran, Jayaraj. et. al. "Curcumin and Cancer Cells: How Many Ways Can Curry Kill Tumor Cells Selectively?." *AAPS J* 11, no. 3 (2009): 495-510.

[377] Zhang. "Curcumin Promotes Apoptosis In Human Lung Adenocarcinoma Cells Through MiR-186* Signaling Pathway." *Oncology reports* 24, no. 5 (2010): 1217-23.

[378] Zhang, Jian, Tao Zhang, Xinyu Ti, Jieran Shi, Changgui Wu, Xinling Ren, and Hong Yin. "Curcumin Promotes Apoptosis In A549/DDP Multidrug-resistant Human Lung Adenocarcinoma Cells Through An MiRNA Signaling Pathway." *Biochemical and Biophysical Research Communications* 399, no. 1 (2010): 1-6.

[379] Clark, CA. et. al. "Curcumin Inhibits Carcinogen and Nicotine-induced Mammalian Target of Rapamycin Pathway Activation in Head and Neck Squamous Cell Carcinoma." *Cancer Prev Res (Phila)* 3, no. 12 (2010): 1586-95.

[380] Quiroga, A, PL Quiroga, E Martinez, EA Soria, and MA Valentich. "Anti-Breast Cancer Activity of Curcumin on the Human Oxidation-Resistant Cells ZR-75-1 with Gamma-glutamyltranspeptidase Inhibition." *J Exp Ther Oncol* 8, no. 3 (2010): 261-6.

[381] Ibrahim, I. et. al. "Effect of Curcumin and Meriva on the Lung Metastasis of Murine Mammary Gland Adenocarcinoma." *In Vivo* 24, no. 4 (2010): 401-8.

[382] Han, Yunkyung, Tomoaki Haraguchi, Sumie Iwanaga, Hiroyuki Tomotake, Yukako Okazaki, Shigeru Mineo, Akiho Moriyama, Junji Inoue, and Norihisa Kato. "Consumption Of Some Polyphenols Reduces Fecal Deoxycholic Acid And Lithocholic Acid, The Secondary Bile Acids Of Risk Factors Of Colon Cancer." *Journal of Agricultural and Food Chemistry* 57, no. 18 (2009): 8587-8590.

[383] Kang, Ju-Hee, Ki-Hoon Song, Jong-Kyu Woo, Myung Hwan Park, Man Hee Rhee, Changsun Choi, and Seung Hyun Oh. "Ginsenoside Rp1 From Panax Ginseng Exhibits Anticancer Activity By Down-regulation Of The IGF-1R/Akt Pathway In Breast Cancer Cells." *Plant Foods for Human Nutrition* 66, no. 3 (2011): 298-305.

[384] He, BC. et. al. "Ginsenoside Rg3 Inhibits Colorectal Tumor Growth Through the Down-Regulation of Wnt/ß-catenin Signaling." *Int J Oncol* 38, no. 2 (2011): 437-45.

[385] Yan, Amy. "Hot Tea or Hot Air? Immunomodulatory Effects of Panax Ginseng in the Prevention of Cancer." *Nutrition Bytes* 4, no. 1 (1998): 1-5.

[386] Sugiyama, T. "Combination of Theanine with Doxorubicin Inhibits Hepatic Metastasis of M5076 Ovarian Sarcoma." *Clin Cancer Res* 5, no. 2 (1999): 413-6.

[387] Zhang, G, Y Miura, and K Yagasaki. "Effects of Dietary Powdered Green Tea and Theanine on Tumor Growth and Endogenous Hyperlipidemia in Hepatoma-Bearing Rats." *Biosci Biotechnol Biochem* 66, no. 4 (2002): 711-6.

[388] Sadzuka, Y, T Sugiyama, and T Sonobe. "Improvement of Idarubicin Induced Antitumor Activity and Bone Marrow Suppression by Theanine, a Component of Tea." *Cancer Lett* 158, no. 2 (2000): 119-24.

[389] Israilides, C., D. Kletsas, D. Arapoglou, A. Philippoussis, H. Pratsinis, A. Ebringerová, V. Hříbalová, and S.E. Harding. "In Vitro Cytostatic And Immunomodulatory Properties Of The Medicinal Mushroom Lentinula Edodes." *Phytomedicine* 15, no. 6-7 (2008): 512-519.

[390] Ng, ML, and AT Yap. "Inhibition of Human Colon Carcinoma Development by Lentinan from Shiitake Mushrooms (Lentinus edodes)." *J Altern Complement Med* 8, no. 5 (2002): 581-9.

[391] Isoda, N. et. al. "Clinical Efficacy of Superfine Dispersed Lentinan (beta-1,3-glucan) in Patients with Hepatocellular Carcinoma." *Hepatogastroenterology* 56, no. 90 (2009): 437-41.

[392] Oba, K, M Kobayashi, T Matsui, Y Kodera, and J Sakamoto. "Individual Patient Based Meta-analysis of Lentinan for Unresectable/Recurrent Gastric Cancer." *Anticancer Res* 29, no. 7 (2009): 2739-45.

[393] Shimizu, K. "Efficacy of Oral Administered Superfine Dispersed Lentinan for Advanced Pancreatic Cancer." *Hepagastroenterology* 56, no. 89 (2009): 240-4.

[394] Jantova, S, L Cipak, and S Letasiova. "Berberine Induces Apoptosis Through A Mitochondrial/caspase Pathway In Human Promonocytic U937 Cells." *Toxicology in Vitro* 21, no. 1 (2007): 25-31.

[395] Serafim, Teresa L., Paulo J. Oliveira, Vilma A. Sardao, Ed Perkins, Donna Parke, and Jon Holy. "Different Concentrations Of Berberine Result In Distinct Cellular Localization Patterns And Cell Cycle Effects In A Melanoma Cell Line." *Cancer Chemotherapy and Pharmacology* 61, no. 6 (2008): 1007-1018.

[396] Mantena, S. K. "Berberine, A Natural Product, Induces G1-phase Cell Cycle Arrest And Caspase-3-dependent Apoptosis In Human Prostate Carcinoma Cells." *Molecular Cancer Therapeutics* 5, no. 2 (2006): 296-308.

[397] Parada-Turska, J. et. al. "Antiproliferative Activity of Parthenolide against Three Human Cancer Cell Lines and Human Umbilical Vein Endothelial Cells." *Pharmacol Rep* 59, no. 2 (2007): 233-7.

[398] Curry III, Eardie A., Daryl J. Murry, Christy Yoder, Karen Fife, Victoria Armstrong, Harikrishna Nakshatri, Michael O'Connell, and Christopher J. Sweeney. "Phase I Dose Escalation Trial Of Feverfew With Standardized Doses Of Parthenolide In Patients With Cancer." *Investigational New Drugs* 22, no. 3 (2004): 299-305.

[399] Zhang, S, C Ong, and H Shen. "Involvement Of Proapoptotic Bcl-2 Family Members In Parthenolide-induced Mitochondrial Dysfunction And Apoptosis." *Cancer Letters* 211, no. 2 (2004): 175-188.

[400] Gao, Xiang, et al. "Prospective Studies of Dairy Product and Calcium Intakes and Prostate Cancer Risk: A Meta-Analysis." *Journal of the National Cancer Institute*, 97, no. 23 (2005): 1768-1777.

[401] Zhu, G, YQ Zhang, and B Wan. "Role of Dietary Factors in Prostate Cancer Development." Zhonghua Nan Ke Xue 11, no. 5 (2005): 375-8.

[402] Larsson, SC, N Orsini, and A Wolk. "Milk, Milk Products and Lactose Intake and Ovarian Cancer Risk: a meta-analysis of epidemiological studies." *Int J Cancer* 118, no. 2 (2006): 431-41.

[403] Chan, JM. et. al. "Dairy Products, Calcium, and Prostate Cancer Risk in the Physicians' Health Study." Am J Clin Nutr 74, no. 4 (2001): 549-54.

[404] Mayo Clinic Staff. "Low White Blood Cell Count." http://www.mayoclinic.com/health/low-white-blood-cell-count/MY00162/DSECTION=causes accessed 30 Aug., 2013.

[405] Sandler, DP, and JA Ross. "Epidemiology of Acute Leukemia in Children and Adults." *Semin Oncol* 24, no. 1 (1997): 3-16.

[406] Mandal, Ananya. "Prostate Cancer Linked to Pesticides: Study." The Medical News. http://www.news-medical.net/news/20110831/Prostate-cancer-linked-to-pesticides-Study.aspx?utm_source=twitterfeed&utm_medium=twitter (accessed March 2, 2012)

[407] Zahm, SH, and WH Ward. "Pesticides and Childhood Cancer." *Environ Health Perspect.* 106, no. 3 (1998): 893-908.

[408] "Chlordane." U.S. Environmental Protection Agency. http://www.epa.gov/ttn/atw/hlthef/chlordan.html (accessed March 5, 2012).

[409] Pogoda, JM, and S Preston-Martin. "Household Pesticides and Risk of Pediatric Brain Tumors." *Environ Health Perspect* 105, no. 11 (1997): 1214-20.

[410] "Alcohol, Tobacco And Breast Cancer – Collaborative Reanalysis Of Individual Data From 53 Epidemiological Studies, Including 58515 Women With Breast Cancer And 95067 Women Without The Disease." *British Journal of Cancer* 87, no. 11 (2002): 1234-1245.

[411] Mulcahy, Nick. "Even Light Alcohol Drinking Ups Breast Cancer Risk: No Safe Level?" http://www.medscape.com/viewarticle/761187 (accessed March 30, 2012).

[412] Stanford University. "Even Low Exposure to X-rays, Gamma Rays Increases Cancer Risk, Study Finds. *ScienceDaily*. 2005, October 27. http://www.sciencedaily.com/releases/2005/10/051027090539.htm (accessed April 1, 2012).

[413] Feychting, M. et. al. "Magnetic Fields and Childhood Cancer–a pooled analysis of two Scandinavian studies." *Eur J Cancer* 31A, no. 12 (1995): 2035-9.

[414] Ahlbom, IC. et. al. "Review of the Epidemiologic Literature on EMF and Health." *Environ Health Perspect* 109, no. 6 (2001): 911-33.

[415] Brouwer, F. P. "Re: "Case-Control Study Of Childhood Cancer And Exposure To 60-Hz Magnetic Fields"." *American Journal of Epidemiology* 141, no. 4 (1995): 375-376

[416] Bethwaite, P, A Cook, J Kennedy, and N Pearce. "Acute Leukemia in Electrical Workers: A New Zealand case-control study." *Cancer Causes Control* 12, no. 8 (2001): 683-9.

[417] Draper, G.. "Childhood Cancer In Relation To Distance From High Voltage Power Lines In England And Wales: A Case-control Study." *BMJ* 330, no. 7503 (2005): 1290.

[418] Gerson Institute. "Dr. Max Gerson" http://gerson.org/gerpress/dr-max-gerson/ accessed September 16, 2013.

[419] Null, Gary. *Get Healthy Now! AComplete Guide to Prevention, Treatment, and Healthy Living*. New York: Seven Stories Press, 1999

[420] Ibid.

[421] Ibid.

[422] Ibid.

[423] Null, Gary. *Get Healthy Now! A Complete Guide to Prevention, Treatment, and Healthy Living*. New York: Seven Stories Press, 2001.

[424] Sodi-Pallares, Demetrio et. al. "A Low Sodium, High Water, High Potassium Regimen in the Successful Management of Some Cardiovascular Diseases: Preliminary Clinical Report." *Can Med Assoc J* 83, no. 6 (1960): 243-257.

[425] Null, Gary. *Get Healthy Now! A Complete Guide to Prevention, Treatment, and Healthy Living*. New York: Seven Stories Press, 1999.

[426] Hildenbrand, G. L., et al. "Five-Year Survival Rates of Melanoma Patients Treated by Diet Therapy after the Manner of Gerson: ARetrospective Review." *Alternative Therapies in Health and Medicine* 1, no. 4 (1995): 29-37. http://www.ncbi.nlm.nih.gov/pubmed/9359807 (accessed March 27, 2012).

[427] Null, Gary. *Get Healthy Now! A Complete Guide to Prevention, Treatment, and Healthy Living*. New York: Seven Stories Press, 1999.

[428] Null, Gary. *Get Healthy Now! A Complete Guide to Prevention, Treatment, and Healthy Living*. New York: Seven Stories Press, 1999.

[429] Ibid.

[430] Gonzalez, Nicholas. *One Man Alone: An Investigation of Nutrition, Cancer, and William Donald Kelley*. New Spring Press, 2010.

[431] Gonzalez, Nicholas, and Linda Isaacs. "The Gonzalez Therapy and Cancer: A Collection of Case Reports." *Alternative Therapies* 13, no. 1 (2007). http://www.alternative-therapies.com/at/web_pdfs/gonzalez1.pdf (accessed April 2, 2012)

[432] Gary Null interview with Dr. Stanley Beyerle. 2/23/95

[433] Chlebowski, RT et. al. "Hydrazine Sulfate Influence on Nutritional Status and Survival in Non-Small-Cell Lung Cancer." *J Clin Oncol* 8, no. 1 (1990): 9-15.

[434] Filov, VA. et. al. "The Results of a Clinical Study of the Preparation Hydrazine Sulfate." *Vopr Onkol* 36, no. 6 (1990): 721-6.

[435] Viegas, Jennifer. "Mistletoe Meds Fight Cancer, Studies Show." Discovery Channel. http://thejourneytogoodhealth.blogspot.com/2012/12/mistletoe-meds-fight-cancer-studies.html (accessed April 1, 2012).

[436] Bar-Sela, Gil. "White-Berry Mistletoe (Viscum album L.) asComplementary Treatment in Cancer: Does It Help?" *European Journal of Integrative Medicine* 3, no. 2 (2011): e55-e62. http://www.europeanintegrativemedicinejrnl.com/article/S1876-3820(11)00024-2/abstract (accessed April 1, 2012).

Index

OKANAGAN REGIONAL LIBRARY
3 3132 03639 4999